CORONARY HEART DISEASE

PRACTICAL CLINICAL MEDICINE

Series Editors J. Fry and G. Sandler

CORONARY HEART DISEASE

Edited by G. Sandler

Consultant Physician
Barnsley District General Hospital
W. Yorkshire

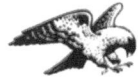 **MTP PRESS LIMITED**
a member of the KLUWER ACADEMIC PUBLISHERS GROUP
LANCASTER / BOSTON / THE HAGUE / DORDRECHT

Published in the UK and Europe by
MTP Press Limited
Falcon House
Lancaster, England

British Library Cataloguing in Publication Data

Coronary heart disease.—(Practical clinical medicine)
   1. Coronary heart disease
   I. Sandler, Gerald   II. Series
   616.1'23   RC685.C6
   ISBN-13: 978-0-85200-940-6   e-ISBN-13: 978-94-010-9218-0
   DOI: 10.1007/978-94-010-9218-0

Published in the USA by
MTP Press
A division of Kluwer Academic Publishers
101 Philip Drive
Norwell, MA 02061, USA

Library of Congress Cataloging in Publication Data

Coronary heart disease.

   (Practical clinical medicine)
   Includes bibliographies and index
   1. Coronary heart disease.   I. Sandler, Gerald,
   1928–   .   II. Series. [DNLM: 1. Coronary Disease.
   WG 300 C8218]
   RC685.C6C644   1986   616.1'23   86–21507
   ISBN-13: 978-0-85200-940-6

Contents

List of Contributors   vi

Series Editors' Foreword   vii

Introduction   ix
     G. Sandler

1   The Management of Heart Attacks   1
     J. R. Hampton

2   The Role of the General Practitioner in the
     Prevention of Coronary Heart Disease   27
     R. Mulcahy

3   Rehabilitation   59
     R. Nagle

4   The Management of Angina   85
     G. Jackson

Index   127

List of Contributors

Professor J. R. Hampton
Department of Medicine
University Hospital
Queen's Medical Centre
Nottingham
NG7 2UH

Dr G. Jackson
Consultant Cardiologist
King's College Hospital
London
SE5 9RS

Professor R. Mulcahy
Cardiac Department
St Vincent's Hospital
Elm Park
Dublin 4
Ireland

Dr R. E. Nagle
Consultant Cardiologist
Queen Elizabeth Hospital
Queen Elizabeth Medical
Centre
Edgbaston
Birmingham
B15 2TH

Series Editors' Foreword

Backing up the pioneering medical researchers and experimenters are the phalanxes and cohorts of practising clinicians in district general hospitals and in general practice who may have to implement and apply any breakthroughs and advances in practical and realistic terms. This they cannot, and should not, be expected to do without careful consideration and analysis. It is essential, therefore, to have regular reviews of the growing points of medicine which are constructively critical as well as being enthusiastic and which can present the issues and implications clearly and fairly to clinicians.

The *Practical Clinical Medicine* series is designed to provide such regular reviews on selected subjects. Each volume is under the charge of an invited editor who selects his team of 4–6 experts. Each contribution is an authoritative, detailed and referenced examination of his topic, is clearly presented in an understandable manner and is practical, relevant and applicable to everyday clinical practice.

The series is intended as a means of communication between researchers and practising clinicians. It is dedicated to generalists who provide primary health care in general practice and to generalists providing secondary medical care in district general hospitals. Both are involved in applying good general practical clinical medicine for their patients, but can only succeed in a climate of constant review and examination.

JOHN FRY
GERALD SANDLER

Introduction

G. Sandler

Coronary heart disease is the largest single cause of death in the UK (1 in 4 of all deaths). Although part of the ageing process, many deaths may be avoidable. The challenges must be how to prevent the condition altogether, how to save lives once it occurs, how to manage complications and how to achieve optimal function in those affected.

Professor Hampton first notes that half of the deaths from myocardial infarction occur suddenly outside hospital when no medical help is possible, and in hospital the overall mortality is 20%. He points out that several trials purporting to show that home care is as good as hospital care were not satisfactory trials and therefore the conclusions unreliable, and considers that the main function of the general practitioner is to get patients into hospital as soon as possible because of the need for resuscitation facilities.

He then goes on to discuss the differential diagnosis of chest pain and points out that a normal ECG does not exclude infarction. He considers that the GP's initial role should be effective pain relief, usually with diamorphine, and readiness for emergency resuscitation at home should cardiac arrest occur.

He discusses the hospital management of myocardial infarction and the complications and seems convinced about the psychological value of a rehabilitation programme.

Beta-blockers are considered desirable for secondary prevention if there is no contraindication, and young patients with ischaemic changes on an exercise ECG after infarction, or those with disabling angina, should be referred for coronary arteriography. Thrombolytic therapy is also discussed.

In conclusion, Professor Hampton reiterates the importance of the GP's role in ensuring early admission and in encouraging return to normal life afterwards.

Professor Mulcahy first emphasizes the 'crucial role' of the general practitioner in primary and secondary prevention of coronary disease and deplores the current preoccupation with cure rather than prevention. He is convinced of the value of controlling the standard risk factors – smoking, hypertension, diet and alcohol – as well as the desirability of altering 'lifestyle', including encouraging exercise.

He goes on to explain the importance of 'face-to-face' health advice given by the practitioner and other health professionals, based on sound scientific knowledge of the risk factors, but stresses the undesirability of burdening patients with controversial views expressed by different doctors.

Professor Mulcahy ends his article by setting out a strategy of prevention to be implemented by the GP including commitment by the doctor, counselling, risk factor screening, health literature, patient's compliance, visual aids and propaganda to highlight unhealthy life habits.

Dr Nagle starts his article by reminding us that the first objective of rehabilitation after a heart attack must be maximum physical recovery and social re-integration into the community; the second aim is to reduce the risk of a further heart attack.

He discusses the adverse effects of prolonged bed-rest and inactivity and the psychological trauma of the heart attack.

He points out the important role of exercise testing in the rehabilitation programme and the value of exercise training.

Finally, Dr Nagle describes the structure and function of his own coronary follow-up clinic at Selly Oak Hospital, the factors which influence recovery after a heart attack and the importance of return to work as a milestone on the path to full recovery.

He concludes that a structured hospital rehabilitation programme is highly desirable after a heart attack and can be provided at relatively low cost.

Dr Jackson introduces his attack on angina with the classic description by Heberden in 1818 which hasn't been bettered. He emphasizes the importance of the history in making the diagnosis and discusses possible examination findings in an anginal patient. He discusses the investigations available – exercise test, nuclear imaging and coronary arteriography – and considers that there is a case for investigating all patients with angina, especially those under 40 years of age, to determine which patients would benefit from coronary artery surgery.

Dr Jackson goes on to stress the importance of primary prevention of coronary disease and emphasizes the role of the general practitioner in discouraging smoking, checking the blood pressure, controlling obesity and encouraging regular exercise.

The specific treatment of angina with nitrates, beta-blockers and calcium antagonists is thoroughly discussed and the place of coronary angioplasty and bypass surgery defined. Dr Jackson then ends his article with a brief account of the mechanism and treatment of unstable angina.

1

THE MANAGEMENT OF HEART ATTACKS

J. R. Hampton

THE DISEASE

'Heart Attack' is a useful term for it encompasses the different manifestations of coronary artery disease. 'Myocardial infarction' is a pathological term used to describe the macroscopic and microscopic changes that are seen in heart muscle that has been deprived of its blood supply for a few hours. The infarction is usually the result of 'coronary thrombosis', but patients can die of a heart attack without a fresh thrombus being demonstrable at autopsy. If a patient dies soon after the onset of symptoms, there may not have been time for the pathological changes of infarction to develop. A patient may die suddenly, usually of an arrhythmia, and a post-mortem examination may demonstrate coronary atheroma but there may be no thrombosis and no infarction. Although the presence of an infarction can be inferred – from the patient's story, his electrocardiogram (ECG) and from changes that occur in serum enzymes – for many clinical purposes it is better to use the old-fashioned term 'heart attack' and to reserve 'myo-

1

cardial infarction' and 'coronary thrombosis' for their proper pathological purposes.

Epidemiology

Heart attacks cause more deaths than any other disease and are by far the most common cause of death in middle aged men. The 'risk factors' for heart attacks are well known. Heart attacks are more common in patients who smoke, who have a high blood pressure, who have a high serum cholesterol, and who are obese. Less important risk factors are a bad family history (death of a parent from a heart attack before the age of 50) and a lack of habitual exercise. Many people, however, have heart attacks without any of these risk factors; and it is important to remember that a risk factor is something associated with an increased risk of a disease but it is not necessarily a cause. Smoking is almost certainly a causal factor – for once an individual stops smoking, his or her increased risk gradually disappears. However, treating high blood pressure does not have any marked effect in preventing heart attacks[1] and there is no convincing evidence that either reduction of serum cholesterol or an increase in exercise have a useful effect.

The death rate from heart attacks has fallen markedly in the USA in the past decade[2]; the death rate used to be much higher than that of the UK, but that of the USA is now similar to that of England and Wales. In England the death rate has probably also started to fall; but it is much higher, and probably constant, in Scotland. The reason for these changes in mortality trends is unknown and is probably not totally explicable by changes in the known risk factors.

Prognosis

Half of the patients who have a heart attack die from it, and half of these deaths occur within two hours of the onset of symptoms[3]. This high early death rate provides the rationale for the immediate management of patients with heart attacks, which will be discussed later. At least half the deaths will occur suddenly, in circumstances where medical help is not available, and the patient who survives long enough to reach hospital represents a selected group. By the time six hours have elapsed from the onset of symptoms, two thirds of the deaths that are going to occur will have done so. Most patients who survive the first 24 hours have an excellent chance of surviving the next week.

The in-hospital death rate – including the whole period from arrival in the accident and emergency department, the period in the coronary care unit (CCU) and the period of convalescence in a medical ward – is about 20%. The death rate is very much higher in old than in young people, and in those who have had previous heart attacks[4].

Mortality rate	
In hospital	20%
1st month after discharge	5–10%
1st year thereafter	5%

In the first month after discharge from hospital, a further 5–10% of patients will die and another 5% will die in the next year[5]. The outlook for the survivors of the acute phase is thus very good, and a patient who leaves hospital has at least an 85% chance of being alive a year later. As the years pass, the excess risk of death gradually declines; and after 10 years, the survivor of a heart attack has much the same risk of death as a person of the same age and sex without any previous history of heart trouble.

THE ROLE OF THE GP

There is an increasing tendency for patients, or their relatives to dial '999' for an emergency ambulance when symptoms of a heart attack occur – for the symptoms are often severe and dramatic. Given the high early death rate, this tendency is to be encouraged; and patients need to be educated to call for help from the emergency services rather than from their GP, for few GPs are equipped to deal with the problems that occur in the early phases of a heart attack. At least half of the patients in an urban area will call an emergency ambulance; though in rural areas, GPs still tend to receive the first call for help[6].

Home care

Three studies published in the 1970's suggested that home care could produce equally good results as could hospital admission[7,8,9]. However, none of these studies was very large, none was a good and simple clinical trial, and all related to the particular sort of patients who called for help from a GP rather than from the ambulance service. In most cases, some four hours had elapsed before the GP accepted responsibility for the patient; and as we have seen, it would be expected that such patients would require much less active management. Despite a considerable amount of local interest, both by GPs and hospital physicians, we now know (unpublished data) that only about 5% of patients who have heart attacks in Nottingham are cared for at home.

Although a GP can quite reasonably keep a patient at home if he or she has delayed calling for help for several hours, or if the journey to hospital is likely to be long and arduous, the main aim of the GP (at least, of the urban GP) is to ensure rapid hospital admission.

The GP will, however, play an important part in the long-term management of surviving patients.

THE PRE-HOSPITAL PHASE OF A HEART ATTACK

Diagnosis

The immediate diagnosis of a patient with a heart attack has to be made on clinical grounds. This is mainly because of the need to get the patient as quickly as possible to a place where resuscitation facilities are available, but also because investigations can be unhelpful and even misleading.

A large minority of patients who have a heart attack will have a previous history of a heart attack or of angina, so when chest pain occurs the diagnosis will immediately be suspected. The pain of a heart attack is usually characteristic: it is central but it radiates to the arm, neck, jaw, teeth, or back.

```
Symptoms in MI
  ● Chest pain
      Radiation:   Arms
                   Neck
                   Teeth
                   Jaw
                   Back
  ● Vomiting
  ● Syncope
  ● Breathlessness
```

It is constant and it is often described as 'crushing' in nature. It is usually severe and is associated with sweating and often with vomiting. There may be associated breathlessness and not infrequently a syncopal episode (either due to a transient tachycardia or to intense vagal-induced bradycardia) will be described.

The physical signs are typically those associated with severe pain. The patient usually lies still and is anxious, cold, and sweaty. There is usually a sinus tachycardia but the pulse rate can be very fast, very slow, or irregular if an arrhythmia occurs. The blood pressure is unhelpful: intense peripheral vasoconstriction may be associated with a high systolic (and sometimes diastolic) pressure; but when the cardiac output is impaired, either by an arrhythmia or by massive cardiac damage, the blood pressure may be low. There may be evidence of heart failure – raised jugular venous pressure, a gallop rhythm at the cardiac apex and moist sounds at the lung bases.

Signs in MI

- Still patient
- Anxious, cold, sweaty
- Sinus tachycardia (but may be slow)
- Blood pressure high or low
- May be heart failure –
  gallop rhythm
  crepitations lung bases
  raised JVP

It should not take more than two or three minutes to take a quick history and to examine the patient for the relevant signs. Then a management decision can be taken. Although an ECG may provide confirmatory evidence of a mycardial infarction, it is not particularly helpful in the early stages because the characteristic changes of infarction may take some hours to develop. About 10–20% of the patients eventually

> Early ECG normal in
> 10–20% of cases

shown to have had an infarction have a normal (or near normal) ECG at the time of admission to a CCU[10]. Unfortunately, this is not always properly appreciated and patients are from time to time inappropriately sent home from accident and emergency departments because of a normal ECG. The only useful role for an ECG in the early phase of a heart attack is to monitor and diagnose the cardiac rhythm (for this it is essential), but unless a GP is able to recognize arrhythmias and treat them, recording an ECG will only delay hospital admission.

Differential diagnosis

Numerous conditions can mimic a heart attack, and these must be borne in mind as the history is being taken and the patient is examined. Patients with many conditions are admitted to CCUs, but this does not matter. The important thing is to ensure that all patients with a heart attack reach a CCU as quickly as possible. Those with other diagnoses can then be sorted out at leisure. The most important conditions to remember are:

(1) Cardiac ischaemia not due to infarction
    A severe attack of angina is one form of 'heart attack' and can be indistinguishable clinically from a myocardial infarction. An immediate distinction is not important. However, if cardiac pain persists for more than 10 or 15 minutes and does not respond to sublingual glyceryl trinitrate, then it can be assumed that the patient has more than angina. It is important to remember that cardiac pain

```
┌─────────────────────────────────────┐
│ Differential diagnosis of chest pain │
│ ● Pulmonary – pleurisy               │
│                infection             │
│                infarction            │
│                pulmonary embolus     │
│                pneumothorax          │
│ ● Aortic dissection                  │
│ ● Pericarditis                       │
│ ● Oesophageal – oesophagitis         │
│                 rupture              │
│ ● Musculo-skeletal                   │
└─────────────────────────────────────┘
```

can result from a primary arrhythmia, such as uncontrolled atrial fibrillation.

(2) *Pain arising in the lungs and pleura*
Pleuritic pain due to infection or infarction can be recognized by the relation to respiration and by the associated cough, sputum production and auscultatory signs. A large central pulmonary embolus can, however, produce chest pain very similar to that of a heart attack. A pneumothorax may cause severe chest pain and collapse, but the pain is usually unilateral.

(3) *Aortic dissection*
Typically, the pain of aortic dissection is described by the patient as 'tearing' in nature and it radiates through to the back. Although peripheral pulses may disappear and the blood pressure may be unequal in the two arms, these are unreliable signs. The appearance of a murmur of aortic regurgitation, particularly if it is associated with a pericardial friction rub, is a strong pointer to the diagnosis of dissection.

(4) *Pericardial pain*
Pericarditis may complicate myocardial infarction. Pericardial pain is typically worse on lying flat and is relieved

by sitting up and leaning forward. It is, however, usually a relatively late complication of infarction and if a pericardial rub is heard early in the illness, pericarditis due to some cause other than infarction is likely.

(5) *Oesphageal pain*
Oesophagitis, usually associated with reflux, can be recognized from the effect of food, posture and alkali. Oesophageal rupture can cause an intense pain that may be confused with that of a heart attack and must be suspected when the pain is preceded by vomiting.

(6) *Musculoskeletal pain*
Pain can radiate round the chest wall from the back when nerve roots are compressed by a vertebral collapse – due to trauma, tumour, myeloma, infection, or osteoporosis. The spine will then usually be tender to percussion. Secondary deposits of tumour in the sternum and ribs can also cause severe pain. Muscle pain can also be confused with cardiac pain and the classical example is the viral infection called 'Bornholm disease' that produces intercostal myositis.

IMMEDIATE MANAGEMENT OF A PATIENT WITH A SUSPECTED HEART ATTACK

The most important part of the management of a patient with a heart attack is pain relief. Strong analgesics are needed and diamorphine (5 mg iv or im) is ideal because it relieves anxiety as well as pain. Diamorphine has the considerable disadvantage for GPs that it is a controlled drug and for those who prefer not to carry such drugs, a proven alternative is buprenorphine (0.3 mg iv)[11]. Buprenorphine can also be given sublingually, although it then has a slightly slower onset of action.

Immediate management
- Pain relief – diamorphine
  buprenorphine
- Bradycardia – iv atropine 0.6 mg
- Tachycardia (> 160/min) – iv lignocaine 100 mg
- Breathless – iv frusemide 40 mg
  sc or im diamorphine

There is no convincing evidence that any drug should be given routinely for prophylaxis – although it is possible that an intravenous beta-blocker, such as metoprolol or atenolol, may cause some reduction of mortality in patients already at low risk[12]. In patients at high risk because of a large infarction, treatment with beta-blockers may theoretically be dangerous. There is no convincing evidence for the routine use of anti-arrhythmic agents, such as lignocaine.

Arrhythmias can only be managed effectively when their nature has been identified by ECG. However, if the patient has a very rapid heart rate (over 160 per minute) and there are signs that the circulation is compromised (the patient is breathless, cold, clammy and hypotensive), the rhythm may well be ventricular tachycardia. If it is, an intravenous injection of lignocaine (100 mg) will often cause reversion to sinus rhythm – and if in fact some other rhythm is present, lignocaine will do no harm. Similarly, atropine (0.6 mg iv) is reasonable treatment for any bradycardia associated with poor cardiac output.

If the patient is breathless because of pulmonary oedema, intravenous frusemide 20–40 mg should be given. Diamorphine is also good treatment for such patients.

However, apart from pain relief, the most important part of immediate management is to decide whether the patient should be admitted to hospital and if admission is indicated, then this should be arranged as soon as possible.

Transport to hospital

Ambulances equipped with defibrillators are now slowly being introduced throughout the United Kingdom[13]. The concept of the 'Mobile coronary care unit' – a special vehicle that handles all the patients with heart attacks – has been shown to be impracticable, but there is no reason why a defibrillator should not form part of the equipment of all emergency ambulances. Ambulance crews can readily be trained in the use of a defibrillator, but whether it is useful to train them in intubation and intravenous fluid and drug administration is more doubtful[14].

Cardiac arrest

General Practitioners should be prepared to manage cardiac arrest, either pending the arrival of a defibrillator-equipped

---

Cardiac arrest
- A – airway clear
- B – breathing
  (artificial respiration)
- C – circulation
  (cardiac massage)

---

ambulance, or during the journey to hospital. Cardiac arrest is recognized when the patient is unconscious and unrousable, when no pulse can be felt and when breathing has ceased. Although as the brain becomes anoxic the pupils will dilate, this is a late sign that indicates brain damage and the diagnosis of an arrest should be made before pupil abnormalities appear. If the 'ABC' rule is followed, a patient with an arrest can be maintained in a viable state (that is, without brain damage) for at least half an hour.

'A' is for airway

False teeth, foreign bodies and vomit must be removed from the patient's mouth. The jaw should be pulled forward and the neck extended (head backwards) to pull the tongue forward from the back of the pharynx. The airway must be kept clear throughout the resuscitation procedure.

'B' is for breathing

Mouth to mouth is the only effective form of artificial respiration. The lungs of the patient should be inflated by four quick breaths at the beginning of the resuscitation attempt and thereafter two breaths should be given between each 11 cycles of cardiac compression.

'C' is for circulation

The circulation is maintained by ensuring that the patient is flat on a firm surface and the sternum is then sharply compressed downwards by about two inches. Compression should be repeated at a rate of about one per second, with 11 compressions between respiratory cycles.

THE HOSPITAL PHASE OF A HEART ATTACK

A major purpose of hospital admission is to ensure adequate pain relief. If the GP elects to keep a patient at home, he must be prepared to visit two or three times during the first 24 hours as repeated analgesic injections may be needed. The second main purpose of hospital admission is to treat complications of infarction. Many patients have no complications and need only one dose of an analgesic, but it is not possible to identify these patients in the early stages.

The most important complications of a heart attack are arrhythmias and heart failure. Less common are venous thrombosis and pulmonary embolism, arterial embolism due to thrombus formation over the infarction in the left ventricle, and pericarditis. A heart attack may directly or indirectly bring to light other problems: diabetes may develop in a susceptible individual due to the stress of the illness; and the use of intravenous diuretics may precipitate urinary retention. Because many patients with heart attacks have other problems and because patients with many diseases can benefit from the special equipment and highly trained staff that have been the characteristic of coronary care units, there is now a tendency to abandon the term 'Coronary care unit' and to substitute 'High dependency unit'. These units handle patients with other problems, such as diabetic ketoacidosis, as well as those with heart attacks.

Arrhythmias

A classical function of a CCU is to monitor the patient's cardiac rhythm, so that ventricular fibrillation or other life-threatening arrhythmias can rapidly be detected and accurately treated. In essence, a CCU is a place where nurses use defibrillators[15]. The practice of the 1960's and 70's was to have one or more nurses continuously watching ECG monitors, but it is now accepted that this is both ineffective and unnecessary[16]. It used to be thought that there were specific 'warning' arrhythmias, which heralded ventricular fibrillation; but it is now known that no arrhythmias provide a useful warning of impending trouble. Ventricular extrasystoles are accepted as one of the indicators that myocardial infarction has occurred and these extrasystoles do not of themselves need treatment.

Any arrhythmia that causes haemodynamic impairment (poor peripheral perfusion, hypotension and heart failure) must of course be treated and since treatment must be preceded by accurate diagnosis, the CCU is still the best place for a patient with a heart attack. Only a minority of patients, however, require such specific treatment.

Heart failure

Diuretics remain the mainstay of the treatment of heart failure. For pulmonary oedema these are combined with amino-phylline (250 mg iv slowly) and diamorphine (5 mg iv). patients who fail to respond may be treated with vasodilators,

---

Heart failure treatment
- diuretic, e.g. frusemide iv 40 mg
- aminophylline iv 250 mg
- diamorphine
- vasodilators
    - sodium nitroprusside
    - iv nitrates

---

the rationale being either to reduce the resistance against which the heart has to pump ('after-load') or to reduce the pressure that fills the heart ('pre-load'). In essence, arteriolar vaso-dilators reduce after-load and venous dilators reduce pre-load. Sodium nitroprusside is a commonly used agent that affects both arterioles and veins – intravenous nitrates predominantly affect pre-load. The accurate use of such drugs is made much easier if the pressure that fills the left ventricle is known; and this is measured by 'floating' a balloon tipped catheter via a vein into the pulmonary artery to measure the pulmonary capillary wedge pressure. This pressure equals that in the left atrium, which in turn is the filling pressure of the left ventricle. This 'Swan Ganz' technique is now commonly used, though it has to be accepted that patients ill enough to need it do not do well, whatever form of treatment they are given.

Other complications

Other complications of myocardial infarction are treated as necessary. Anticoagulants are usually only given pro-phylactically to patients who are at special risk of venous thrombosis – this includes those with heart failure, who may be confined to bed for more than the usual period. Pericarditis can be treated with indomethacin. Occasionally patients develop catastrophic problems – such as myocardial rupture, rupture of the interventricular septum and severe mitral regurgitation due to papillary muscle rupture – and although these are usually fatal, occasionally the lives of such patients can be saved by prompt open heart surgery.

Other complications of MI
- risk of DVT – anticoagulants
- pericarditis – indomethacin
- surgery for – myocardial rupture
  ruptured inter-
  ventricular septum
  papillary muscle
  rupture

Bed rest

There is no need for a patient to remain in bed longer than he wants to, and as soon as the pain has settled a patient should be up[17]. ECG monitoring can be maintained by telemetry, and patients gain a considerable psychological uplift from being allowed up and from losing their 'umbilical' attachment to an ECG monitor.

The duration of hospital stay

Most patients remain in a CCU for 24–48 hours and are then transferred to a medical ward. Here they are allowed up and are encouraged to walk about. They should be fully mobile after 5 or 6 days. Patients who have no complications needing specific treatment (the majority) can safely be discharged home after a week in hospital.

THE POST-HOSPITAL PHASE OF A HEART ATTACK

Although most patients are well by the time they leave hospital and require little or no specific treatment, the GP has a vital role to play in helping the patient to overcome the psychological trauma inevitably associated with a heart attack. Relatives and well-wishers often try to persuade the patient to 'take things easy' and generally retire to bed and become an invalid. There is no evidence at all that this is beneficial, and the GP must ensure that it does not happen.

There is no evidence either that supervised exercise programmes prolong life or promote early return to normality, though there is no doubt that the increase in physical fitness that they induce brings a sense of well being. Much the same effect can be induced by simple encouragement. For example, a patient should be told to go for a walk twice a day and to increase the distance daily. A month after the heart attack, the patient should be able to walk a mile at a normal speed. The patient should be encouraged to resume a normal sex life as soon as he feels like it.

Return to work

Most patients should be able to return to work after a month, although with the current employment problem and the opportunities for early retirement many men are now not working again after a heart attack. Any one who has had a myocardial infarction is not permitted to hold a heavy goods vehicle or public service vehicle driving licence ever again, and this regulation deprives many patients of their livelihoods. Return to work may be delayed because patients should be advised not to drive for at least two months: this is partly to allow the main risk period to pass, and partly so that a patient will have learned to recognize and deal with an attack of angina before he starts driving[18].

For all these 'non-medical' reasons, many patients who have had a heart attack do not return to work after a month, but this should remain the aim.

Of course there are some medical reasons why people cannot return to work so quickly and some patients will have sufficiently severe angina or heart failure to make it impossible for them to carry out their job. Heavy jobs are relatively unusual these days, but patients with heavy work may need a rather longer period of convalescence and exercise, and it is prudent for them to return to light work first (if possible).

The follow-up of heart attack patients

There is no necessity for routine exercise testing or coronary angiography in patients who have recovered from a heart attack, though both have their place[19].

In some centres all patients have a treadmill test before leaving hospital. At one time it was thought that useful prognostic information was provided by the amount of ischaemic ST segment depression that exercise induced, but it is now accepted that only the pumping action of the heart (indicated by the exercise-induced changes in heart rate and blood pressure) are of prognostic significance[20]. An early treadmill test does not produce information necessary for any particular clinical action, but a later test (perhaps at one or two months) might suggest the need for coronary angiography if ischaemic changes occur at low exercise levels.

Coronary angiography is always indicated if a patient has disabling angina which is not adequately controlled by medical treatment, and coronary artery bypass grafting may be needed for symptomatic relief. It must be remembered, however, that angina tends to improve after a heart attack – and in any case, the risks of surgery are relatively high early on. It is therefore prudent not to embark on coronary angiography

Indications for coronary arteriography
- Inadequate control of angina with drugs
- Main left coronary artery disease
- ? Multivessel disease

with a view to surgery because of angina until two or three months have elapsed.

There remains some doubt whether coronary artery bypass grafting prolongs life, so in a patient with little or no angina angiography is not mandatory[21]. The operation prolongs life in patients with significant narrowing of the main left coronary artery and probably also in patients with proximal disease in all three main arteries, when there is also poor left ventricular function. For milder arterial disease, however, the benefit in terms of longevity is less certain. The risk and morbidity of operation have to be set against any reduction in mortality that a successful operation might achieve; and it has to be remembered that 50% of vein grafts are occluded within 7–10 years, so a patient cannot be offered a 'once and for all' operation.

A reasonable course of action is for all young patients (say, under 55) to have an exercise test after one or two months and for angiography to be performed on those whose ECGs show ischaemic changes at low exercise levels.

Treatment of late complications of infarction

The late complications of myocardial infarction are the same as those that occur in the hospital phase – pain, heart failure and arrhythmia.

At least one third of patients who have a myocardial infarction will have angina afterwards. Glyceryl trinitrate (0.5 mg sublingually) remains the mainstay of treatment, and patients should be encouraged to use as many tablets as necessary and to take them prophylactically before any exertion that might cause angina. Because of their effect on later mortality (see below) any post-infarct patient with angina should be treated with a beta-blocker unless there is a specific contraindication to the use of these drugs, such as asthma or severe heart failure.

Treatment of angina
- Sublingual glyceryl trinitrate
- Betablocker – timolol 10 mg bd
              atenolol 50–100 mg daily
- Ca^{2+} antagonist – nifedipine 10–20 mg tds
- Isosorbide mono/di-nitrate
- Bypass graft if medical treatment fails

If angina is not adequately controlled by trinitrate plus either timolol (10 mg bd) or atenolol (50–100 mg daily) then a calcium antagonist should be added – such as nifedipine 10 mg tds or 20 mg bd if the slow release form is used. Long acting nitrates (isosorbide dinitate 10 mg tds, or isosorbide mononitrite 20 mg bd) can be added if the combination of a beta-blocker and a calcium antagonist proves ineffective. If the simultaneous administration of all three drugs is inadequate, then coronary artery bypass grafting must be considered.

Many patients with heart attacks who develop mild heart failure during their hospital admission are discharged on diuretics, which are frequently unnecessary in the medium or long term. If the patient is well, the only way to find out whether or not the diuretic is helping is to discontinue it. This should be done at one month. If breathlessness or ankle swelling recur, then bendrofluazide 5 mg daily is the best initial treatment. If this proves ineffective, the patient should be changed sequentially to a thiazide–amiloride combination tablet (Moduretic 1 tds) and then to frusemide 40 mg, 80 mg or, if necessary, 120 mg daily. Frusemide should be accompanied by a potassium-retaining diuretic, such as amiloride 5–10 mg

daily. If the patient remains symptomatic despite treatment
with frusemide 80 mg daily, it is essential to consider whether
the heart failure is due to some potentially operable problem –
such as a left ventricular aneurysm, a ventricular septal defect,
or mitral valve regurgitation.

Arrhythmias of all sorts are common following myocardial
infarction but tend to settle with the passage of time. When
complete heart block complicates acute infarction temporary
pacing may be needed, but permanent pacing is necessary in

Long-term arrhythmia treatment

• Supraventricular tachycardia – beta-
                                  blocker
                                  verapamil
• Atrial fibrillation – digoxin
• Ventricular tachycardia – flecainide

---

only 5% of these patients. Tachyarrhythmias must be treated
if they cause symptoms and the nature of the arrhythmia
should be established before treatment is commenced. Atrial
fibrillation is best treated with digoxin, supraventricular tachycardias with a beta-blocker or verapamil and ventricular tachycardias with flecainide.

THE SECONDARY PREVENTION OF HEART ATTACKS

'Secondary prevention' is the term used to describe the prevention of further heart attacks in a patient who has already
had one. 'Primary prevention' means preventing a first attack.
The risk factors that are associated with an increased chance
of a first attack are much less important for long term survival
in a patient who has recovered from a first heart attack,
perhaps because survival is mainly controlled by the amount
of heart muscle that has been destroyed. Reduction of serum
cholesterol is unhelpful for secondary prevention and there is

no certain evidence that reduction of blood pressure or weight reduces the risk of subsequent heart attacks – though both are important for other reasons. Smoking, however, remains an important risk factor and stopping smoking undoubtedly reduces the risk of a second, as well as a first attack. Once the patient returns home from hospital, persuading a patient to stop smoking is the most useful thing a GP can do.

Many trials have been conducted of drugs which, in theory, should prevent later death in patients who have survived a heart attack. In the 1960s and 70s interest was centred on the anticoagulants[22] (Dindevan and later Warfarin). Although there was a fairly consistent trend in the different trials favouring active treatment, no individual trial provided conclusive evidence that such therapy was useful. One of the most persuasive studies was reported from Holland[23], where patients who had been anticoagulated for several years after a heart attack were randomly allocated to groups in which treatment was either continued or stopped. The patients who continued fared better – but of course this does not necessarily prove that they should have been treated in the first place.

Since many deaths from heart attacks occur suddenly due to ventricular fibrillation, it might be supposed that prophylactic administration of an anti-arrhythmic agent would be beneficial. In fact this is not so and drugs like mexiletine and disopyramide confer no benefit[24, 25]. Such drugs do prevent ventricular extrasystoles and ventricular tachycardia; but it is not clear whether their failure to improve survival stems from an inability to prevent ventricular fibrillation, or occurs because the drugs are actually harmful. It is quite possible that this is so, for all antiarrhythmic drugs may induce heart failure and most of them can actually induce arrhythmias in some patients.

Twenty years ago beta-blockers were first tested in the survivors of heart attacks – in the largely misplaced belief that they had powerful anti-arrhythmic properties[26]. After numerous trials, there can now be no doubt that routine treatment with a beta-blocker is beneficial after a heart attack. Although reduction of mortality in such patients may well be a general property of all the drugs of this type, it is not clear in all cases what dose should be used. The evidence is best for timolol 10 mg bd[27] or propanolol 80 mg bd[28], and one of these should be prescribed. Precisely *when* treatment should begin is not clear: soon after a heart attack beta-blockers may induce heart failure, but if treatment is delayed too long some patients who might have been helped will die before they are treated. Two weeks after the attack is probably the right time to start and treatment should be continued for two years.

Ideally, beta-blocker treatment would be given only to those patients with a substantial risk of death or reinfarction, but in fact these drugs do benefit patients of all risk categories and it is easiest to prescribe them routinely. It is perfectly reasonable to discontinue them in low risk patients (those who are young and who have had a first, small infarction) if unacceptable side effects occur.

Secondary prevention
- Stop smoking
- Beta-blockers

FUTURE TRENDS IN HEART ATTACK MANAGEMENT

The therapy that seems at present to have the greatest potential is thrombolysis. The body's natural defence against thrombosis is the fibrinolytic system, in which a plasma protein called plasminogen is activated to the enzyme plasmin, which destroys fibrin. Activation of the fibrinolytic system can undoubtedly 'dissolve' fresh thrombi in coronary arteries and angiographic studies suggest that 70–80% of occluded arteries can be re-opened, provided that treatment is begun within four hours of the onset of symptoms. The best-known activator of fibrinolysis is streptokinase, but this has the disadvantage of destroying fibrinogen as well as fibrin and can therefore cause hazardous bleeding. Two new plasminogen activators are more specific for fibrin in thrombi and these should be less hazardous. These compounds are a streptokinase–plasminogen complex and a synthetic version of the natural tissue plasminogen activator, which is now produced by genetic engineering techniques[29].

It is still not known whether thrombolytic treatment will prolong life. Even when a thrombus has been lysed, an atheromatous plaque will remain in the coronary artery and rethrombosis may occur quite soon. It may be that balloon dilatation (angioplasty) or coronary artery bypass grafting will have to be performed if any early benefit of thrombolysis is to be maintained.

Thrombolytic therapy is only effective when commenced early and if it does prove life-saving, it will become all the more necessary to educate patients and their relatives to summon help quickly when chest pain occurs.

Practical points

- Patients with suspected heart attacks are best admitted to hospital, especially if seen soon after the onset
- Relief of pain is main objective in an uncomplicated attack
- A beta-blocker should be used for secondary prevention
- After discharge GP should encourage a quick return to normal life (unless there are serious complications, e.g. heart failure)
- Stopping smoking is the most important part of both primary and secondary prevention

CONCLUSIONS

Heart attacks are common and are frequently fatal, though the long term prognosis of those who survive the acute phase is very good. If a patient has chest pain, which may be a heart attack, the GP's main role is to ensure rapid admission to hospital whenever possible. On the patients return home, the GP must encourage a quick return to normal life. Management of an uncomplicated attack is essentially simple and consists of pain relief during the acute phase and prophylactic treatment with a beta-blocker later. Persuading people to stop smoking is the most important part of both primary and secondary prevention.

REFERENCES

1. Medical Research Council Working Party (1985). MRC trial of treatment of mild hypertension: principal results. *Br. Med. J.,* **291,** 97–104
2. Hampton, J.R. (1982). Falling mortality in coronary heart disease. *Br. Med. J.,* **284,** 1505–6
3. Fulton, M., Julian, D.G. and Oliver, M.F. (1969). Sudden death and myocardial infarction. *Circ.,* **40** (Suppl. 4), 192–5
4. Wilcox, R.G. and Hampton, J.R. (1980). Importance of age in prehospital and hospital mortality of heart attacks. *Br. Med. J.,* **44,** 503–7
5. Wilcox, R.G., Roland, J.M. and Hampton, J.R. (1981). Prognosis of patients with 'chest pain. ? cause'. *Br. Med. J.,* **282,** 431–3
6. Hill, J.D., Hampton, J.R. (1976). Mode of referral to hospital of patients with heart attacks: relevance to home care and special ambulance services. *Br. Med. J.,* **2,** 1035–1036
7. Mather, H.G., Pearson, N.G., Read, K.L.O., *et al.* (1971). Acute myocardial infarction: Home and hospital treatment. *Br. Med. J.,* **3,** 334–8
8. Hill, J.D., Hampton, J.R., Mitchell, J.R.A. (1978). A randomised trial of home–versus–hospital management for patients with suspected myocardial infarction. *Lancet,* **1,** 837–41
9. Colling, A., Dellipiani, A.W., Donaldson, R.J., MacCormack, P. (1976). Teeside coronary survey: an epidemiological study of acute attacks of myocardial infarction. *Br. Med. J.,* **2,** 1169–72.
10. McGuinness, J.B., Begg, T.B., Semple, T. (1976). First electrocardiogram in recent myocardial infarction. *Br. Med. J.,* **2,** 449–51

11. Hayes, M.J., Fraser, A.R., Hampton, J.R. (1979). Randomised trial comparing buprenorphine and diamorphine for chest pain in suspected myocardial infarction. *Br. Med. J., 2*, 300–2.
12. Hjalmarson, A., *et al.* (1981). Effect on mortality of metoprolol in acute myocardial infarction. *Lancet, 2*, 823–6
13. Jones, R.H. (1983). Management of cardiac arrest in the community: a survey of resuscitation services. *Br. Med. J., 287*, 968–971
14. Thompson, R.G., Hallstrom, A.P. and Cobb, L.A. (1979). Bystander-initiated cardiopulmonary resuscitation in the management of ventricular fibrillation. *Ann. Intern. Med., 90*, 737–740
15. Lown, B., Fakhro, A.M., Hood, W.B. and Thorn, C.W. (1967). The coronary care unit. *J. Am. Med. Assoc., 199*, 156–166
16. Vetter, N.J., Julian, D.G. (1975). Comparison of arrhythmia computer and conventional monitoring in coronary-care unit. *Lancet, 5*, 1151–1161
17. Hayes, M.J., Morris, G.K. and Hampton, J.R. (1974). Comparison of mobilization after two and nine days in uncomplicated myocardial infarction. *Br. Med. J., 3*, 10–13
18. Medical aspects of fitness to drive. A guide for medical practitioners. (London: Medical Commission on Accident Prevention)
19. Epstein, S.E., Palmeri, S.T. and Patterson, R.E. (1982). Evaluation of patients after acute myocardial infarction. Indications for cardiac catheterization and surgical intervention. *N. Engl. J. Med., 24*, 1487–1492
20. Jennings K., Reid, D.S., Hawkins, T., Julian, D.J. (1984). Role of Exercise testing early after myocardial infarction in identifying candidates for coronary surgery. *Br. Med. J., 288*
21. Hampton, J.R. (1984). Coronary artery bypass grafting for the reduction of mortality: an analysis of the trials. *Br. Med. J., 289*, 1166–1170
22. Mitchell, J.R.A. (1981). Anticoagulants in Coronary heart disease – retrospect and prospect. *Lancet, 1*, 257–62
23. Report of the Sixty Plus Reinfarction Study research group (1980). A double-blind trial to assess long-term oral anticoagulant therapy in elderly patients after myocardial infarction. *Lancet, 2*, 980–994
24. Wilcox, R.G., Rowley, J.M., Hampton, J.R., Mitchell, J.R.A., Roland, J.M., Banks, D.C. (1980). Randomised placebo-controlled trial comparing oxprenolol with disopyramide phosphate in immediate treatment of suspected myocardial infarction. *Lancet, 2*, 765–69
25. Chamberlain, D.A., Julian, D.G., Boyle D.McC., Jewitt, D.E., Campbell, R.W.F., Shanks, R.G., *et al.* (1980). Oral mexiletine in high-risk patients after myocardial infarction. *Lancet, 2*, 1324–1327
26. Snow, P.J.D. (1965). Effect of propranolol in myocardial infarction. *Lancet, 2*, 551–553
27. The Norwegian Multicentre Study Group. Timolol-induced reduction in mortality and reinfarction in patients surviving acute myocardial infarction (1981). *N. Engl. J. Med., 304*, 801–807
28. Co-operative Trial: Preliminary Report. The Beta-blocker heart attack trial (1981). *J. Am. Med. Assoc., 246*, 2073–2074

29. Randomised trial of intravenous recombinant tissue-type plasminogen activator versus intravenous streptokinase in acute myocardial infarction. Report from the European Co-operative study group for Recombinant Tissue-type Plasminogen Activator (1985). *Lancet*, **1,** 842–847

2

THE ROLE OF THE GENERAL PRACTITIONER IN THE PREVENTION OF CORONARY HEART DISEASE

R. Mulcahy

INTRODUCTION

The Royal College of General Practitioners issued two recent documents as part of an initiative to improve and transform certain aspects of general practice[1,2]. One area which demands a greater commitment by general practitioners is the promotion of health among their patients and the prevention of the common chronic diseases in the community.

Traditionally, and because of the education doctors receive at undergraduate and postgraduate levels, we are more concerned with the treatment of sick people than with the maintenance of health and a healthy society. We can identify and measure our therapeutic successes but our success in prevention will pass unnoticed – at least by our individual patients.

Current medical education has failed to keep pace with changes in the pattern of disease over the past one or two generations and has failed to take note of the crucial role of the general practitioner in the fields of primary and secondary prevention. The lack of interest in and the lack of commitment to preventive medicine are the rule rather than the exception among physicians today. The very structure and organisation of our hospitals and our health services, combined with an almost exclusive preoccupation with the treatment of ill people, discourage a preventive approach.

Public interest in prevention

We must see the situation in the context of what is happening around us. There is an increasing groundswell of interest in prevention among the public. Already quite dramatic changes are taking place in certain countries and among certain social and professional classes. These changes have already led to a dramatic reduction in the incidence of chronic diseases such as coronary heart disease, stroke and hypertensive heart disease[3, 4]. Doctors are one social group which has greatly reduced cigarette smoking, with a consequent reduction in mortality from lung cancer and coronary heart disease[5].

Public interest in the prevention of disease is increasing and the pressures on doctors and politicians to provide more information and better facilities to maintain natural health is apparent in most of our communities.

Britain has been slower than most countries in responding to the evidence that we can now prevent coronary heart disease, stroke and other vascular conditions by simple lifestyle changes and by the control of cigarette smoking and alcohol abuse. The rather poor professional and public response to preventive exigencies in Britain may reflect the failure of epidemiologists to present convincing and consensus evidence of the causes of coronary heart disease and of the implications of their impact on the public health.

While the incidence of coronary heart disease in the United Kingdom may now be falling[6], the British record compares very unfavourably with those of the United States, Canada, Australia, New Zealand and Finland. These and other countries are showing falls in mortality from coronary heart disease of more than 20% during the last 15 years[3, 4, 7]. In some cases the fall in mortality is as high as 35% and in one case, Australia, it is now reported that mortality from coronary heart disease may be down by a massive 50%[8, 9].

The case for prevention

Controversy still continues about the efficacy and the desirability of adopting preventive measures at a population level. This controversy is probably more evident and more active in the United Kingdom than in most other countries. Some epidemiologists and physicians are too rigid in the criteria of evidence they demand before approving a public health and educational programme. They believe that dietary change and hypertension control, among other interventions, must be shown to be unequivocally effective before appropriate lifestyle changes should be recommended. Incontrovertible proof of benefit is not available and is never likely to be available as regards such interventions – mainly because of the logistic difficulties inherent in the large population trials which would be necessary to satisfy these rigid criteria.

In my view, by demanding proof that desirable changes in lifestyle could not lead to harmful results, some colleagues are unnecessarily cautious. For example, some experts in the field of hypertension believe that a reduction of salt level to 5.0 g a day may have harmful results[10]. At a public health level, this is an unacceptable view, since 5.0 g is well above the minimum physiological requirement of sodium chloride and some com-

munities with such low levels of salt intake have good health
records[11].

The clinical, epidemiological and basic research evidence
that appropriate dietary changes, control of hypertension, the
cessation of smoking, the greater use of exercise and the control
of alcohol abuse, will benefit the public health is so compelling
that it would be negligent of us not to advise appropriate and
desirable lifestyle changes at a personal and community level.
The dramatic secular changes in mortality from coronary heart
disease and stroke in America, Australia and other countries
are entirely consistent with the changes in lifestyle which are
occurring there; and are consistent with the basic, experi-
mental, epidemiological, clinical and pathological research
that identified the primary risk factors – smoking, diet, and
hypertension – as having a causative role in the genesis of

Desirable changes in life-style
- Dietary changes
- Control of hypertension
- Stopping smoking
- Control of alcohol excess

---

atherosclerosis and coronary heart disease. There is clear evidence in these countries that the fall in mortality can be
attributed to a reducing incidence more than to improved case-
fatality rates because of better treatment[7]. Research should
continue into the risk factor background of coronary heart
disease and, where there are gaps in our knowledge or some
issues are undecided, debate and controversy must continue
within the profession. It is wrong, however, that such controversies should be allowed to obscure the need for the public
to adopt a healthier lifestyle. With the current knowledge of
risk factors, the public can and should take full responsibility
for personal and family health, based on commonsense and
the consensus views of many independent and authoritative
bodies – such as the Surgeon General of The United States,

the DHSS, the World Health Organisation, the International Society and Federation of Cardiology and the Royal College of Physicians.

The natural history of coronary disease

It is worth looking at the pattern of disease that exists in current society. Most diseases are chronic and come to our attention when they present with an acute exacerbation. They are then usually at an advanced stage. This is characteristic of the pattern of coronary disease. Most patients currently admitted to coronary care with myocardial infarction will have advanced atherosclerosis. Most will be ignorant of coronary risk factors. They will usually be discharged without adequate counselling and advice about the control of such risk factors, despite the fact that there is increasing evidence that risk factor modification after a coronary attack reduces the risk of subsequent sudden death or death from myocardial infarction or other non-coronary causes[12].

It is a feature of the common chronic diseases that the number of risk factors that are operative is relatively limited. Smoking, alcohol abuse, unhealthy diet, obesity, lack of exercise and possibly stress, constitute most of these. These risk factors are related to multisystem disease and the interaction of risk factors can produce a variety of apparently unrelated clinical conditions, which account for the common phenomenon of clustering of disease in our patients. Many people go through life without significant illness and reach a normal biological lifespan. Others admitted to our hospitals and seen in general practice show a clustering of disease. Duodenal ulcer, bronchitis, arterial disease, arthritis, gout, diabetes, chronic obstructive lung disease, hypertension and premature ageing may exist in various combinations in a surprising number of middle-aged individuals. We should not think of coronary disease in terms of single cause and effect[13].

While my purpose is to discuss the prevention of coronary

disease in this paper, I am aware that such a concept is unrealistic and too narrow. If we succeed in preventing coronary heart disease, we shall also make great strides in the prevention of many other chronic conditions – including stroke, peripheral vascular disease, bronchitis and emphysema, lung cancer, bladder cancer, duodenal ulcer, diabetes, hypertension and gout. Therefore, when we are adopting a strategy of prevention and a positive health programme in general practice, although we may be particularly concerned about the prevention of coronary heart disease and stroke, we must also be conscious of the great power and potential we possess to prevent other conditions by encouraging natural health, a good quality of life and the prevention of premature ageing. This comprehensive concept of prevention is a satisfying one and is certainly a rational and logical approach, which may help to achieve the WHO ideal, adopted in the declaration of Alma-Ata, with its lofty aspiration of *Health for all by the year 2000*[14].

The role of the general practitioner

General practitioners, more than any other group of professionals, are qualified to fulfil a major role in improving the standards of public health by becoming involved in counselling their patients about the principles of natural health. It has been shown that doctors in face-to-face interviews are more influential than any other people in persuading patients to stop smoking[15]. Their intervention is more effective than other widely adopted techniques, such as smoking clinics, nicotine chewing gum and hypnotism. The advice of a general practitioner dedicted to health promotion, particularly when well informed about the scientific basis of prevention, can be effective in having patients adopt the necessary behavioural changes aimed at achieving a life of natural health. General practitioners see most of their patients every year[16]. If every smoking patient attending were given counselling advice (requiring a brief two or three minutes) backed up by appropriate literature, within a few years there would be a substantial reduction in cigarette smoking in these islands.

Advice need not necessarily be given by the doctor. Other health professionals can be just as effective, but the perceived support of the doctor and the doctor's commitment to a health

---

Advice about smoking
- The patient must want to stop
- The patient must be well informed about:
    The smoking related diseases
    The benefits of stopping
- Stopping suddenly is more effective than stopping gradually
- The smoker must build up a sustained conflict about the habit
- Withdrawal effects should be anticipated and explained

---

maintenance programme will have a powerful added influence. Doctors in particular should be more concerned with a positive health approach, not only because of our privileged position and our greater knowledge, but also because most of us have adopted the healthier lifestyle that needs to be advocated. There has been a remarkable reduction in smoking among doctors in Britain[5] and, if we are to judge by recent trends in mortality within the medical profession compared to the general population, most of us have adopted effective measures to protect our own personal health. It seems that, *noblesse oblige,* we should share our good fortune with our patients and with the public.

I have been practising primary and secondary preventive medicine as part of my normal clinical and consultation work for many years. I find that many patients are eager to learn the principles of positive health. With proper counselling and example, they will frequently adopt recommended behavioural changes. The practice of clinical preventive medicine is a very satisfying one. It adds a new dimension to our work, and a new meaning and fulfilment to the doctor/patient relationship. We must conceive of medical practice at its best as a combination of health promotion and maintenance, disease prevention, treatment and continuing care[16].

It is perhaps easier for the hospital physician to be involved in preventive medicine because of the availability of staff and facilities, and the longer duration of consultations. However, I believe the same service can be given by the general practitioner.

If doctors and other health personnel hope to influence patient behaviour – aimed at the promotion of positive health and the prevention of coronary heart disease – it is essential that their advice should rest on a knowledge of the scientific basis of risk factors. A profound knowledge of the clinical, research and epidemiological evidence is not necessary but we should be aware of the principal evidence supporting an association between risk factors and disease. We should be familiar with some of the consensus opinions proferred on diet and smoking by commissions or working parties appointed by national or international agencies. In our discussion with patients it is futile and divisive to expound in detail about the various controversial aspects of causation and intervention. Such controversies are better confined to a professional milieu; or at least, if they are stated in public, our uncertainties and doubts should not lead to confusion among the public about the basic principles of health promotion. Unless there are important conceptual changes as regards aetiology, brought about by new research findings, we should accept the advice of suitably qualified expert groups on the question of causation and intervention.

CORONARY RISK FACTORS

I would like to deal in a little detail with some of the risk factors that are deemed to be important in maintaining the present high level of coronary heart disease in this country.

Hyperlipidaemia

A high mean national cholesterol level is the dominant risk factor for coronary heart disease[17]. No country with a high mean cholesterol level has a low incidence of coronary heart

The management of hypercholesterolaemia	
Total cholesterol (mmol/l)	*Action*
< 5.5 mol (210 mg%)	Normal balanced diet Avoid excess of saturated fat
5.5–6.4 (211–240 mg%)	Limited intake of saturated fat
6.5–7.4 (241–280 mg%)	Strict saturated fat and cholesterol limitation
7.5 (281 mg%)	If persistent in two or more readings, and not responding to diet, interrupted courses of cholestyramine

disease. Low incidence countries such as Japan have mean levels of 150–160 mg% (3.91–4.14 mmol/l) among middle-aged males, while high incidence countries have levels of between 220 or 230 mg% (5.70–5.93 mmol/l). It is likely that the biological normal level of cholesterol is close to 160 mg% (4.14 mmol/l) and that we should be more rigid in our interpretation of the accepted norm in the western world.

The clinical, pathological, basic research and epidemiological evidence linking high saturated fat diet with high mean levels of cholesterol and with a high incidence of coronary heart disease is so persuasive and so consistent[18] that we cannot afford to ignore the importance of balanced and appropriate diet in the prevention of heart disease. Action is compelling when we recall that at least 40 national or international commissions are unanimous in advocating a reduction in the level of saturated fat consumption and in the mean cholesterol level of the population[19]. Some of these commissions also favour: a reduction in cholesterol-rich food; an increase in coarse carbohydrate and high fibre foods; and, in certain circumstances, an increase in the intake of polyunsaturated fats.

Simple dietary changes can normalize the hyperlipidaemia associated with the modern lifestyle of excessive saturated fat intake, lack of exercise and overweight[20]. An appropriate balanced diet can be more varied and enjoyable, and just as economical, as the traditional Northern European diet. Dietary change does require some change in culinary methodology but those of us who have already made these changes are aware that the new cooking techniques are simple and easily adopted.

Evidence about diet as a major factor in aetiology of coronary heart disease has been ably presented by Stuart Truswell[19, 21]. His papers are important reading for those concerned with the dietary aspects of heart disease prevention.

Hypertension

There is little controversy about the need to control established hypertension. The aim should be to bring blood pressure down to normal or near normal levels. However, there is still uncertainty about how we should manage hypertension, particularly in relation to the use of drugs and the use of non-pharmacological methods of control. We still lack conclusive evidence that control of hypertension will reduce the risk of heart attack in primary prevention studies, although some trials have shown benefit[22]. There is only slim evidence that control will be effective in the secondary prevention of coronary disease[23, 24]. However, there is persuasive evidence that control of established hypertension is beneficial in preventing stroke, left ventricular failure, renal failure and rupture of aneurysm[22]. It is mandatory therefore that high blood pressure should be identified and properly controlled.

Non-pharmacological control of BP
- Salt restriction
- Regular exercise
- Control of obesity
- Limitation of alcohol intake
- Stress avoidance
- Relaxation techniques

Non-pharmacological methods of control are important. These include salt limitation, regular and adequate exercise, the control of obesity, limitation of alcohol and the avoidance of excessive stress. Bio-feedback and relaxation techniques have also been recommended. It is likely that mild or borderline hypertension can be controlled by non-pharmacological methods. Indeed, drug therapy may be contraindicated in mild hypertension because of side-effects, which may adversely affect prognosis.

Because of the high incidence of borderline hypertension, and the cost and undesirable side-effects of drugs, it is essential that the population control of mild hypertension should be along physiological and natural means. With close cooperation between the doctor and patient, drugs may be used intermittently to deal with any exacerbations of high blood pressure but in many cases non-pharmacological methods will suffice.

It is not my purpose to discuss the merits of the various drugs that are available, but clearly we need careful judgement in their employment. We must avoid preparations that cause intolerable side-effects and may cause complications or aggravate other risk factors. Relevant examples are the adverse effects of thiazide diuretics on the lipid profile, on glucose metabolism and on uric acid metabolism. The negatively inotropic effect of beta-blockers may further impair the function of a damaged left ventricle.

Our own case history study of patients with myocardial infarction confirms that hypertension is a frequent finding in both males and females with coronary heart disease[25, 26]. As a risk factor, hypertension tends to operate in middle-aged and older people – unlike cigarette smoking, which dominates the risk factor scene in younger patients and particularly in those under 50 years of age.

Cigarette smoking

There is little argument about the role of cigarette smoking as a cause of multiple system disease. It is the greatest single cause of premature mortality and of chronic illness in our society[27]. Cessation of cigarette smoking is unequivocably beneficial in both primary and secondary studies of coronary heart disease[27, 28].

Doctors in these islands have largely eschewed the smoking habit. It seems therefore that we are sharing our good fortune with our patients when we advise them to stop smoking. Informed and unequivocal counselling by a general practitioner has been shown to be the most effective way of getting people to stop[15].

If we are asked by our patients about the evidence linking cigarette smoking with coronary heart disease, we can cite the numerous and detailed reports issued by the Surgeon General of the United States over the past 21 years[27].

We may also be asked about mechanisms. The nicotine absorbed by the inhaling cigarette smoker stimulates catecholamine production – thus increasing blood pressure, heart rate and the irritability of heart muscle. Nicotine may also affect platelet fragility and adhesiveness, and may have a thrombogenic effect[29, 30].

The inhaled carbon monoxide in cigarette smoke adversely

affects the oxygen-carrying function of haemoglobin, thus reducing the amount of oxygen available to the myocardium. It may also affect the utilisation of oxygen at the cellular site. Carboxyhaemoglobin and nicotine, and possibly other inhaled

Effects of smoking	
Nicotine	• Increased catecholamines:
	Increased BP
	Tachycardia
	Myocardial irritability
	Thrombotic tendency
	Platelet damage
Carbon monoxide	• Reduced O_2 in blood
	• Reduced cellular uptake O_2
	• Myocardial irritability
	• ? Increases atherosclerosis

constituents, have complex metabolic and arrhythmogenic effects but no clear consensus has yet been reached about the role of these constituents in the genesis of atherosclerosis and coronary heart disease[27].

There is, however, clear evidence from basic research studies that the adverse effects of cigarette smoking are enhanced by and possibly dependant on the presence of hyperlipidaemia[27]. This is consistent with the epidemiological findings that communities and countries with low mean serum cholesterol levels (such as Japan) have a low incidence of coronary heart disease, despite the fact that the smoking habit may be widespread[31].

Obesity

There is little evidence that obesity is an independent risk factor for coronary heart disease but it increases susceptibility to hypertension, diabetes, hyperlipidaemia, arthritis and many other conditions. It is also more frequently associated with sudden death[32]. The lifespan of the obese is shortened.

Control of obesity is a difficult and complex problem. Compliance to advice is often poor. Crash diets seldom succeed. We need to enquire about the cause of overeating in our patients and there is much evidence that satisfactory longterm control can only be achieved by regular supervision and counselling, occasionally by psychotherapy and by adopting vigorous and aerobic exercise. The assistance of a dietitian will help, but dietetic services are seldom available outside hospital. Longterm adherence to a balanced and moderately low calorie diet with more bulk food, combined with longterm commitment to physical activity with a good aerobic component, offers the best hope.

Stress

There is much popular support and not a little professional support for the concept that stress is an important risk factor for coronary heart disease. While acute stress may precipitate a life-threatening or fatal arrhythmia in a susceptible person with coronary artery disease, there is little evidence that chronic stress is an important primary cause of atherosclerosis and coronary heart disease. However, careful counselling aimed at relief of stress is an important part of our professional work if we are to alleviate our patients medical and psychological problems.

The over-ambitious, dynamic and work-addicted patient has been called a Type A personality[33]. This personality type is considered by a minority of researchers to be a primary coronary risk factor. This contention is difficult to confirm, but there is evidence that some people can be taught to change their personalities and adopt a more relaxed and detached attitude to life. To do this, it may be necessary to seek the assistance of a psychologist or a trained counsellor, but most members of a cardiac rehabilitation staff can be trained to discuss and alleviate stress and can succeed in altering some of the characteristics of the Type A personality. Indeed, such counselling is also the essence of good doctoring.

The prevention of coronary heart disease
- Regular aerobic exercise
- Ensure blood pressure is normal
- A balanced diet – restrict red meats, high fat dairy and processed foods
- No cigarette smoking, no inhaling of other tobacco
- Know your blood pressure and cholesterol levels

Family history

There are wide differences of opinion about the importance of family history in coronary heart disease[34, 35]. While there is nothing we can do about our genetic origin, we should be aware that risk factors – such as smoking, unhealthy diet, hypertension and lack of exercise – tend to aggregate in families. I believe this aggregation of risk factors is the principal, if

Family risk factors
- Smoking
- Hypertension
- Lack of exercise
- Unhealthy diet
- Hypercholesterolaemia

not the only, cause of the high frequency of coronary heart disease in certain families. Patients presenting with a positive family history should be carefully screened for risk factors. If absent, these patients can be fully reassured and advised that they are at low risk for coronary attack.

THE STRATEGY OF PREVENTION IN GENERAL PRACTICE

A practical preventive programme requires attention to the following strategies:

- Knowledge of risk factors and commitment by the doctor
- Counselling
- Screening
- Health literature
- Visual aids, including posters, figures or tables, presenting data on causation and prevention
- Suitable devices to confirm and highlight the influence of unhealthy life habits.

Professional commitment

Commitment by the doctor is an essential part of primary and secondary prevention in general practice. As previously stated, a committed doctor will be more influential in achieving desirable lifestyle changes than any other intervention methods. To be effective, however, we must have knowledge of the scientific basis of risk factors so that we can speak with some conviction and authority to our patients and to other health personnel.

Counselling

Advice and counselling by the well-informed health professional is the basis of the preventive strategy. A few minutes counselling by the doctor will be effective but his influence will be enhanced if the practice nurse or even the receptionist can be involved in the counselling process. The part-time or full-time practice or district nurse may be encouraged to advise patients about personal lifestyle, to advise about family health, to carry out simple screening procedures and to distribute

---

Counsellors
- Doctor
- Practice nurse
- District nurse
- Health educationalist (local authority)
- Dietition
- Social worker

---

appropriate literature. We find nurses to be excellent counsellors in our hospital rehabilitation service and in our primary preventive work in the Irish Heart Foundation. They are easy to motivate and train, and in Britain they can be engaged at little or no extra cost to the family doctor. The general practitioner who employs a nurse will have 70% of her salary paid by the National Health Service. Tax relief will be granted on the residual 30%. If you employ a nurse for 10 hours – long enough to help in counselling, screening and to do other things besides – it will cost you £7 a week but will make your life easier and will also contribute to the improvements in general practice, which are recommended by the Royal College of General Practitioners[1, 2].

You can also make use of the services of a facilitator to help you plan a preventive strategy and to train your nurses in health promotion and screening[36]. The service of a facilitator should be sought through your local health authority.

With a little initiative, the family doctor should be able to employ part-time or full-time health personnel to widen the scope of general practice and to introduce a really worthwhile preventive component. The reader is referred to published works that will assist in planning an effective prevention programme[15, 37].

Screening

The merits and feasability of screening for early disease (pre-symptomatic screening) give rise to much controversy, but there can surely be no differences of opinion about the need to carry out simple risk factor screening as part of routine family doctoring. Every patient attending a general practitioner should have a blood pressure check at first visit. The frequency of further checks depends on the patient's blood pressure status. Even in normotensives the blood pressure should be measured at least every three years.

Weight is easy and quick to measure, while the question of a cholesterol check may pose greater difficulties. If all patients accepted advice to follow a healthy balanced diet, it should not be necessary to carry out routine cholesterol checks. However, there are circumstances in which at least one cholesterol measurement should be arranged:

- Patients over 25 years at their first visit
- Patients with a positive family history for coronary disease or stroke
- Patients with a history of a high fat intake
- Overweight and sedentary patients
- Those with coronary risk factors including smoking, hypertension and diabetes
- Those who are anxious to ascertain their lipid status.

Patients with other coronary risk factors, such as hypertension and smoking, are at greater risk if the serum cholesterol is raised. Their motivation to change lifestyle may be reinforced by knowing their cholesterol level. A simple serum cholesterol measurement suffices in most cases. It is cheap and does not require fasting beforehand.

We need to be more strict in interpreting normal levels of cholesterol. As stated earlier, the mean national levels among middle-aged males in these islands, where the population is at high risk for coronary heart disease, is considerably higher than the mean level in populations at low risk, such as Japan.

Therefore in Britain, the mean level should not be considered an ideal or normal level. The Japanese level may be the biological norm and perhaps we should be aiming at these levels or close to them for our own population. However, it would seem reasonable – at this relatively early stage of public health intervention – to aim at levels under 200 mg% (5.2 mmol/l).

Draconian dietary measures are not necessary to achieve a substantial reduction in serum cholesterol levels. Satisfactory reductions may be achieved by relatively simple changes, which need cause little hardship or inconvenience.

If cholesterol levels are excessively high, say above 250 mg% (6.5 mmol/l), it may be necessary to order a complete lipogram – including triglycerides and high density lipoprotein cholesterol – if such facilities are locally available. Stricter dietary measures may be required for a limited period of time in those with high levels; while chemotherapy, in the form of the ion-exchange resin cholestyramin, may be necessary as a temporary or permanent measure in more severe cases. Ideally, a lipid clinic and laboratory should be available in every hospital region to provide assistance in the management of the more severe and intractable hyperlipidaemias.

Health literature

Appropriate health literature should be freely available in the surgery and waiting room. If a general practitioner or physician gives a health leaflet to a patient at risk and encourages him to read it, then re-read it and, if necessary, to come back to discuss its contents, the patient will not infrequently respond. Appropriate health literature, particularly in relation to the prevention of heart disease, is available from the Coronary Prevention Group, the British Heart Foundation, the DHSS, the Chest and Heart Association, The Health Education Council and local health authorities.

Please ask to have your name put on the mailing list of these organisations and ensure that they send you adequate supplies.

It is surprising how avidly patients avail themselves of this literature, particularly if it is personally presented by the doctor. The doctor's signature on the literature will add to his authority.

Visual aids

Appropriate posters and visual health data are also available from some voluntary as well as local and central health authorities. They can be displayed in the waiting room or surgery. They too have a valuable influence, particularly with the less educated patients who will respond more readily to the visual message rather than to the written word.

Other devices and procedures

Simple procedures and devices may be employed to emphasise the health message and to bring home to patients the need to make simple lifestyle changes. The weighing machine and the sphygmomanometer are familiar to us. A peak flow meter can be informative about the adverse effect of smoking on pulmonary function and, in hospital practice, measurement of carbonmonoxide in exhaled air by a desk oximeter gives immediate and impressive information about the quantity of smoking and depth of inhalation. Simple coronary risk factor calculators are becoming more freely available and will stimulate the interest and participation of patients. You should enquire about these from the Coronary Prevention Group, the British Heart Foundation or the Health Education Council.

FAMILY HEALTH

General practitioners are also intimately concerned with family health. It is here that health promotion will achieve its greatest benefits over the longterm. Breast milk is less atherogenic than cow's milk, particularly where the mother has a low saturated fat intake. A balanced family diet, with a reduction in the present high levels of saturated fat and with an increase in carbohydrates, should be prescribed for the

---

Family health points
- breast milk better than cow's milk
- balanced family diet – less saturated fat
                             increase in
                             carbohydrate
                             No free salt on table

---

whole family. A minute or two with the housewife or parent may be sufficient to ensure a healthy diet policy for the family. Young parents who have one or two young children are particularly likely to respond to counselling in this area.

Salt should not be available on the table. By this means children will not acquire the taste for salt. Eating between meals by children and the eating of convenience or 'junk' food should be discouraged, particularly if we are to counteract the tendency to obesity in the young population.

There is little doubt that atherosclerosis starts in childhood, as is confirmed by the relative frequency of the condition found in autopsies[35].

PATIENT ATTITUDES AND OTHER FACTORS AFFECTING COMPLIANCE

We must be realistic about our patient's ability to respond to the advice we proffer. While lifestyle advice by a doctor is more effective than any other method of intervention, we must recognize the greatest challenge in achieving successful primary and secondary prevention – the capacity of our patients to comply with our advice. Compliance is influenced by a number of personal, psychological and environmental

Advice on secondary prevention

- No tobacco
- Balanced diet with limitation of saturated fat/high cholesterol foods. Limitation of calories if necessary
- Control hypertension by non-pharmacological and, if necessary, pharmacological means
- Encourage regular aerobic exercise and physical fitness
- Encourage early return to normal active life without routine restrictions

factors. Education, social background, personality and personal relationships all play a part in determining a patient's commitment to behavioural change. These factors must be recognized and indeed they are probably appreciated by the general practitioner more than by doctors in hospital practice or elsewhere. Good compliance to advice is not easy to achieve, particularly over the longterm; but it is undoubtedly a more likely prospect if the doctor and his staff are seen to be committed and dedicated to the patient's welfare and if lifestyle advice is based on rational and practical lines.

Desired behavioural change is made easier under the following circumstances:

- The patient and family must be fully informed about the nature of the problem
- Social and family support may be necessary
- Repeated counselling
- Appropriate literature
- Good communication with health professionals
- Patient involvement with management.

Patient involvement in management is by no means a new concept. For many years it has ensured a high degree of success in the management of diabetes. The efficient control of diabetes would be impossible without patient self-management. The same techniques could and should be applied to the management of hypertension. Patients in a few Dublin hospitals are taught to take their own blood pressure[39]. They are supplied with a relatively simple and suitable sphygmomanometer at cost price and they are instructed to keep a health diary, in which they record regular blood pressure readings and other details of weight and medication, where appropriate. Hypertension is an area where poor compliance, both as far as non-pharmacological methods and drug therapy are concerned, is notoriously bad. Self-monitoring of blood pressure and optimum involvement of the patient in management has, in our own experience, a dramatic effect on compliance. We believe the principles of self-management and of having patients fully informed about their condition should be adopted by the medical profession more widely.

It is still believed and frequently stated that informing patients about their illness may make them anxious and more insecure. This concept is quite untenable and one has only to talk to the well-informed and well-managed diabetic to know that full and accurate information reduces anxiety and increases motivation. It ensures good management and good adherence to advice. It has always been my experience that full and accurate information provided to patients will be appreciated and will contribute to good longterm care. There are, of course, certain patients who are less receptive to information and who have less interest in knowing about their medical status. Clearly, we must use our discretion when we decide how much information we need to provide.

SECONDARY PREVENTION AND CORONARY HEART DISEASE

Secondary prevention of coronary heart disease is an aspect of prevention which concerns the general practitioner as well as the hospital physician. The aim of secondary prevention is to reduce the risk of non-fatal and fatal myocardial infarction, sudden death, and complications such as heart failure and life-threatening arrhythmias in patients with angina pectoris and in survivors of myocardial infarction.

Secondary prevention may also require longterm and repeated counselling and supervision. However, while compliance still poses a real difficulty in this situation, patients are more likely to respond to our advice because they may perceive themselves as being in a life-threatening situation.

Secondary prevention includes all management techniques, including risk factor modification, drug treatment, coronary artery bypass surgery and angioplasty. It also includes the anticipation, prevention and appropriate management of complications following myocardial infarction. While much publicity and attention is paid to surgery, the use of drugs and the treatment of complications to improve survival, little attention is paid to the importance of risk factor modification and desirable behavioural changes in the coronary patient. Yet, in my view, a comprehensive risk factor modification programme may be more important in improving survival and the quality of life than the combined modalities of surgery and drug treatment.

Risk factor intervention

It is necessary to place considerable emphasis on the need to identify and eliminate coronary risk factors in our patients. This may require desirable lifestyle changes which must be included in a secondary prevention programme.

There are no large randomized control trials of the effect of comprehensive risk factor modification on prognosis and myocardial infarction, apart from one study by Kallio and his colleagues[12]. This study confirms that smoking control and dietary intervention significantly reduced total mortality and

---

Effects of risk factor modification after MI

- Further non-fatal and fatal infarction and sudden death reduced
- Less post-infarction angina
- Other vascular accidents reduced
- Less morbidity and mortality from non-vascular diseases
- Relieves anxiety about further infarction and sudden death

Risk factor modification is an essential part of good cardiac rehabilitation

---

sudden death in survivors of myocardial infarction over a three year period.

There is, however, unequivocal evidence that eliminating cigarette smoking after myocardial infarction confers major benefits in terms of reduced morbidity and mortality[40]. A reduction in the incidence of post-infarction angina in the first six years of follow-up has also been reported[41].

While there is only limited evidence that treating hypertension after infarction will confer benefit in terms of further coronary attack, there is unequivocal evidence that such treatment will reduce the incidence of stroke, left ventricular failure, renal failure and rupture of aneurysm[22]. Adequate treatment of hypertension is therefore essential as part of a secondary prevention programme, particularly in patients with healed infarction who are more susceptible to develop left ventricular failure in the presence of poorly controlled high blood pressure.

A number of workers have tested the effect of dietary control on serum lipids and subsequent prognosis in survivors of myocardial infarction[42]. None of these trials were adequate in design, in numbers of subjects and endpoints, and in length of follow-up, to give meaningful results. None can therefore be considered convincing, but the majority showed some improvement in prognosis.

It would seem logical that we should reduce raised cholesterol levels, at least by simple and physiological dietary means. It is my practice to put all coronary patients on a routine balanced diet with some reduction in saturated fat. In the case of severe hyperlipidaemia, a stricter low saturated fat and low cholesterol regime is required, with the use of continuous or interrupted cholestyramine in the more severe cases.

We have been practising risk factor modification for 20 years as part of our hospital rehabilitation programme. We have learned that simple and repeated counselling of the patient and family can be highly effective in achieving desirable lifestyle changes.

Other aspects of secondary prevention

The prevention and treatment of complications following myocardial infarction is an important part of secondary prevention. The management of post-infarction arrythmias is a complex and rather contentious issue, and will not be dealt with in this article. Drug treatment has to be chosen with care and must be used with discretion because of undesirable side-effects in some patients, but there is no doubt that some preparations may be valuable and life-saving in those who are prone to life-threatening arrythmias. The identification and management of such arrhythmias is usually a matter for the cardiologist, who has the experience and the appropriate facilities available for investigation and who should be consulted as necessary.

Left ventricular failure is a frequent complication and one which may occur quite unexpectedly many months after the patient has fully recovered. It should be anticipated in patients with extensive infarction, in those who are symptomatic and in those with associated conditions that may put an added strain on the left ventricle. These include aortic valve disease, poorly controlled hypertension and a propensity to paroxysmal tachyarrythmias. Left ventricular failure should be anticipated and prevented by attention to associated conditions and by the routine use of diuretics, with or without the use of digitalis or other inotropes.

The management of post-infarction angina depends on the elimination of risk factors, the prescription of appropriate exercise programmes and the use of nitrates, beta-blockers or calcium antagonists to increase the pain threshold and thus facilitate an exercise programme.

There is still considerable controversy about the use of drugs with the primary aim of improving survival. Claims have been made for a variety of medications, including anticoagulants, beta-blockers, the calcium antagonists and the platelet-active drugs, aspirin, sulfinpyrazone and dipyridamole. It would not be possible to include a review of this complex subject in this paper but the reader is referred to the latest consensus opinion of the International Society and Federation of Cardiology published in 1984[43]. This aspect of secondary prevention has been the subject of many other review articles.

Secondary prevention is an essential part of cardiac rehabilitation. Coronary rehabilitation has undergone a major change in direction over the past 20 years. Unlike the cautious and conservative approach to management, which was the rule in earlier years, we now aim to have patients out of bed and out of hospital quickly, and we encourage active exercise programmes and an early return to normal life and to normal work. With proper management and particularly with appropriate and healthy lifestyle changes, patients should perceive themselves as being perfectly normal people who can resume a normal place in family life and in society. Change of occupation is seldom necessary, except in the case of drivers of public service vehicles.

Prohibitions about returning to normal activities should be discouraged and traditional advice about adopting lighter work and avoiding household, sexual and work activities are most inappropriate. Such advice should be confined to the relatively rare patient with severely impaired left ventricular function.

CONCLUSION

The prevention of heart disease in our community is an important public and political issue and is the responsibility of every member of the community. General practitioners, in particular, are in a powerful position to change lifestyle behaviour and to influence the public health through precept and example.

The standing of the general practitioner remains high in our society. It will be assured of remaining so if we are committed to encouraging positive health among our patients.

REFERENCES

1. Irvine, D. (1983). Quality of care in general practice: our outstanding problem. *J. Coll. Gen. Practice,* **33**, 521–3
2. Royal College of General Practitioners, (1985). *Towards quality in general practice: A Council consultation document.* (London: Royal College of General Practitioners)
3. Editorial (1983. Why has stroke mortality declined. *Lancet,* **1**, 1195
4. Marmot, M.G. (1984). Lifestyle and national and international trends in coronary heart disease mortality. *Postgrad. Med. J.,* **60**, 3–8
5. Doll, R. and Peto, R. (1976). Mortality in relation to smoking: Twenty years observation on male British doctors. *Br. Med. J.* **2**, 1525–36
6. Simpson, V. (1984). Trends in major risk factors. Cigarette smoking. *Postgrad. Med. J.,* **60**, 20–5
7. Pell, S. and Fayerweather, W.E. (1985). du Pont de Nemours and Company, Wilmington, DE. *N. Engl. J. Med.,* **312**, 1005–11
8. *National Heart Foundation of Australia, Information Paper No. 19* (1984) (Brisbane: National Heart Foundation of Australia)
9. Goodwin, R. (1985). Personal communication
10. Brown, J.J., Lever, A.F., Robertson, J.I.S., Semple, P., Bing, R.F., Heagarty, A.M. et al., (1984). Salt and Hypertension. *Lancet,* **2**, 456
11. Prior, I.A.M., Evans, J.G., Harvey, H.P.B., Davidson, F. and Lindsey, M. (1968). Sodium intake and blood pressure in two Polynesian populations. *N. Engl. J. Med.,* **279**, 515–20
12. Kallio, V., Hamlaienen, H., Hakkila, J. and Ruurila, O.J. (1979). Reduction in sudden deaths by a multifactorial intervention programme after acute myocardial infarction. *Lancet,* **2**, 1091–4

13. Hickey, N. (1985). The Aetiology of coronary heart disease: implications for the family doctor. *Ir. Med. J.*, **78,** 291–2
14. World Health Organisation. Alma-Ata 1978. Primary Health Care. Report of the International Conference on Primary Health Care, Alma-Ata, U.S.S.R. 'Health for All' Series No. 1. (Geneva: WHO)
15. Rose, G. and Hamilton, P.G.S. (1979). A randomised control trial of the effect on middleaged men of advice to stop smoking. *J. Epidemiol. Community Health,* **32,** 275–81
16. Fowler, G. (1984). The challenge of prevention. *The Practitioner,* **228,** 1143–7
17. Blackburn, H. and Jacobs, D. (1984). Sources of the diet-heart controversy: Confusion over population versus individual correlations. *Circ.* (Editorial), **70,** 775–80
18. Shekelle, R.B., Macmillan, S.A., Paul, O., Leppler, M. and Stamler, J. (1981). Diet, serum cholesterol and death from coronary heart disease. *N. Engl. J. Med.,* **304,** 65–70
19. Truswell, S. (1981). Diet and coronary heart disease – how much more evidence do we need? *Nutr. Bull.,* **6,** 93–107
20. Graham, I., Reid, V., Hickey, N., McFarlane, R., Daly, L., Ruane, P. and Mulcahy, R. (1981). Longterm dietary control of Type II hyperlipidaemia. *Ir. Med. J.,* **73,** 470–2
21. Truswell, A.S. (1985). Reducing the risk of coronary heart disease. *Br. Med. J.,* **291,** 34–7
22. Hypertension Detection and Follow-up Program Coooperative Group. (1979). Five year findings of the hypertension detection and follow-up program. Mortality by weight, sex and age. *J. Am. Med. Assoc.,* **242,** 2572–7
23. Graham, I.M., Mulcahy, R., Hickey, N. and Daly, L. (1978). The effect of hypertension and its treatment on prognosis after myocardial infarction. In Hjalmarson, A. and Wilhelmsen, L. (eds.) *Acute and longterm medical management of myocardial ischaemia,* pp. 279–84. (Molndal, Sweden: Lindgren and Soner)
24. Connolly, D.C., Elveback, L.R. and Oxman, H.A. (1983). Coronary heart disease in residents of Rochester, Minnesota, 1950–1975. 111. Effect of hypertension and its treatment on survival of patients with coronary artery disease. *Mayo Clin. Prog.,* **58,** 259–64
25. Mulcahy, R., Hickey, N. and Maurer, B. (1969). Coronary heart disease: A study of risk factors in 400 patients under 60 years. *Geriatr.,* **24,** 106–14
26. Mulcahy, R., Hickey, N. and Maurer, B. (1967). Coronary heart disease in women: Study of risk factors in 100 patients less than 60 years of age. *Circ.,* **36,** 577–86
27. *The health consequences of smoking: Cardiovascular disease* (1983). Report of the Surgeon General (Rockville, Maryland: DHSS)
28. Mulcahy, R. (1983). Influence of cigarette smoking on morbidity and mortality after myocardial infarction. *Br. Heart J.,* **49,** 410–5
29. Mustard, J.F. and Murphy, E.A. (1963). Effect of smoking on blood coagulation and platelet survival in man. *Br. Med. J.,* **1,** 846–9

30. Horwitz, O. and Waldorf, D.S. (1960). Effects of tobacco smoking on the clotting process in man as measured by thrombelastography. *Circ.*, **22**, 765 (abstract)
31. Keys, A. (ed.), (1980). *Seven countries: Multivariate analysis of death and coronary heart disease.* pp. 136–60. (Cambridge: Harvard University Press)
32. Kannel, W.B., Doyle, J.T., McNamara, P.M., Quickenten, P. and Gordon, T. (1975). Precursors of sudden coronary death. Factors related to incidence of sudden death. *Circ.*, **51**, 606–13
33. Rosenman, R.H., Brand, R.J., Sholtz, R.L. and Friedman, M. (1976). Multivariate prediction of coronary heart disease during 8.5 year follow-up in the Western Collaborative Group Study. *Am. J. Cardiol.*, **37**, 903–10
34. Conroy, R., Mulcahy, R., Hickey, N. and Daly, L. (1985). Is a family history of coronary heart disease an independent coronary risk factor? *Br. Heart J.* **53**, 378–81
35. Friedlander, Y., Kark, J.D. and Stein, Y. (1985). Family history of myocardial infarction as an independent risk factor for coronary heart disease. *Br. Heart J.* **53**, 382–7
36. Fullard, E.M., Fowler, G.H. and Gray, M. (1984). Facilitating prevention in primary care. *Br. Med. J.*, **289**, 1585–7
37. Gray, M. and Fowler, G. (1983). *Preventive medicine in general practice.* (Oxford: Oxford University Press) (In Press)
38. Strasser, Th. (1982). Erforschung and Bekampfung der Arteriosklerose in Kindesalter. *M 'schr. Kinderheilk.*, **130**, 740–2
39. Fitzgerald, D.J., O'Callaghan, W.G., O'Brien, E., Johnson, H., Mulcahy, R. and Hickey, N. (1985). Home recording of blood pressure in management of hypertension. *Ir. Med. J.*, **78**, 216–18
40. Mulcahy, R. (1983). Influence of cigarette smoking on morbidity and mortality after myocardial infarction. *Br. Heart J.*, **49**, 410–15
41. Daly, L.E., Graham, I.M., Hickey, N. and Mulcahy, R. (1985). Does stopping smoking delay onset of angina after infarction? *Br. Med. J.* **291**, 935–7
42. Mulcahy, R., Hickey, N. and Graham, I. (1981). The importance of risk factor control in the secondary prevention of coronary heart disease. In: Wilhelmsen, L. (ed) *Improvements of prognosis of myocardial infarction.* Proceedings of symposium at 8th European Congress of Cardiology. (New York: Academy Professional Information Services)
43. Pyorala, K., Rapaport, E., Konig, K., Schettler, G. and Diehm, C. (eds) (1983) *Secondary prevention of coronary heart disease.* Workshop of International Society and Federation of Cardiology (Stuttgart, New York: Thieme Verlag)

USEFUL ADDRESSES

British Heart Foundation
102 Gloucester Place
London
W1H 4DH

01-935 0185

Health Education Council
78 New Oxford Street
London
WC1A 1AH

01-631 0930

(D.G. Dr David Player)

Action on Smoking and Health
5–11 Mortimer Street
London
W1N 7RJ

01-637 9843

(D.G. David Simpson)

Coronary Artery Disease Research Association (CORDA)
Tavistock House North
Tavistock Square
London
WC1H 9TH

01-387 9779

The Chest Heart and Stroke Association
Tavistock House North
Tavistock Square
London
WC1H 9TH

01-387 3012

(D.G. Sir David Atkinson)

Scottish Health Education Group
Health Education Centre
Woodburn House
Canaan Lane
Edinburgh
EH10 4SG

031-477 8044

ASH (Scottish Branch)
Royal College of Physicians
9 Queens Street
Edinburgh
EH10 4SG

031-447 8044

(D.R. Mrs Alison Hillhouse)

3

REHABILITATION

R. Nagle

INTRODUCTION

Originally used to describe the restoration of rank and privilege to a subject deprived of them by way of punishment, the term rehabilitation was first used in medicine in the fields of orthopaedics and trauma surgery. It implies a recognition of the fact that a patient whose disease has been 'cured' may yet remain disabled and unable to work by reason of direct and indirect consequences of the disease and its treatment. Thus bone disease may give rise to deformity – even when the cause has been eradicated – and immobilization may lead to wasting, weakness and a decline in general health – even though it may be a necessary part of the original treatment. Various kinds of physiotherapy have traditionally played an important part in rehabilitation together with occupational therapy, retraining for a more suitable job and attention to the psychological effects of organic disease.

Rehabilitation in cardiac disease has a much shorter history, but the ideas and principles are the same. Many patients who have survived the dangers of acute heart disease, in particular myocardial infarction, remain disabled, inactive, anxious and unemployed. At the same time, studies of the effects of physical activity on the cardiovascular system have shown that physical training is beneficial to patients as well as to athletes. Rest and physical inactivity, which were once thought of as an important part of the treatment of heart disease, have come under suspicion as risk factors in the causation of disease. Studies of the factors causing delayed recovery have shown that non-organic, psychological factors and non-medical social factors are as important as the heart disease itself in determining the outcome.

Objectives of cardiac rehabilitation

1. The best possible recovery, not only in physical terms but in psychological and social aspects too

Although these three aspects are obviously linked by the effects of the disease, they also have an independent significance of their own.

Objectives of rehabilitation
- Physical recovery
- Psychological acceptance
- Social adaptation –
    return to normal life
    return to productive life
- Reduce risk of recurrence

A common mistake is to assume that a patient who has made a good physical recovery will automatically return to normal life and productive work. There is abundant evidence that psychological disturbances after infarction bear little relationship to the physical severity of the illness. Just why this should be so is far from clear. The knowledge of having been close to death, fear of recurrence and the influence of family and friends with the same fears are probably the main factors. A diagnosis of coronary disease carries social and medico-legal implications, which are also largely independent of the severity of the illness. Someone who drives a bus or lorry will lose their job and anyone unemployed will find it even more difficult to obtain one.

2. To minimize the risk of recurrence of infarction

The traditional risk factors become of less importance once infarction has occurred. Stopping smoking is the only step that has been shown to be of definite benefit. For younger patients, dietary advice designed to normalize abnormal lipids will often be sought and should be provided.

There is no evidence that *routine* coronary angiography (to detect left main stem or multivessel disease) and coronary bypass surgery (in appropriate cases) is of benefit after infarction, but some patients will have severe residual coronary disease and require this treatment. There is good evidence that exercise testing is an effective method of screening for these potentially operable patients and identifying those who require angiography. Patients suffering from disabling heart failure after infarction should be likewise investigated for reparable defects – such as ventricular aneurysm, mitral incompetence and ventricular septal defect.

Methods

Cardiac rehabilitation describes all the measures that help to resolve these different problems. As such, it is considered by many to be no more than a part of good general medicine, but in practice the best results have often been obtained when special attention has been given to this aspect of heart disease and special arrangements made to pursue and co-ordinate the different aspects of treatment.

Rehabilitation may be useful in all forms of heart disease, but it has been studied most intensely in the case of myocardial infarction and it is principally in this context that it will be considered here.

Success in medical treatment is often gauged by the discharge of a live patient from hospital and the need for rehabilitation is often not appreciated by those who fail to follow up the patient into the convalescent stage. Nevertheless, research carried out all over the world has shown that varying degrees of avoidable and unnecessarily prolonged invalidism are common[1, 2]. The earlier studies must be judged against the general background of medical opinion at the time they were made. Twenty years ago, six weeks bed rest and three months restricted activity were commonly prescribed for myocardial infarction and this inevitably led to prolonged inactivity and lengthy periods off work. The elaborate and costly rehabilitation hospitals and rehabilitation programmes set up in parts of Europe must be seen against this background of a conservative medical policy forbidding physical activity in the acute phase of the illness.

The idea that convalescent patients should be encouraged to exercise rather than to rest was a new one and therefore properly applied with caution and rather elaborate precautions[3]. As the benefits of exercise have become more widely recognized and the hazards have proved to be slight, physical training programmes have become simpler and cheaper and have been employed at progressively earlier stages in convalescence.

At the same time the treatment of acute myocardial infarction itself has undergone great changes (especially for the mild case), with a much shorter time in hospital and much earlier mobilization. As a result, it seems likely that the need for formal rehabilitation may be rather less now than it was in the past, since patients are quickly discharged from hospital.

FACTORS INFLUENCING RECOVERY FROM MYOCARDIAL INFARCTION

The risk factors associated with *a liability to develop coronary heart disease* are well known. They are smoking, hypercholesterolaemia and hypertension together with a number of other less definite and less well established factors – such as

> **Risk factors in coronary disease**
>
> - Smoking
> - High cholesterol
> - High blood pressure
> - ? Lack of exercise
> - ? Type A personality

lack of exercise and certain personality traits. The factors determining *prognosis and life expectancy* after a myocardial infarct are very different. At this stage in the disease, prognosis becomes largely determined by the extent of coronary atheroma and the damage that the muscle of the heart has sustained during the myocardial infarction.

Myocardial damage

Heart failure and clinical or radiological evidence of cardiac enlargement are associated with a reduced expectation of life, delayed recovery and inability to work. These risk factors share a dependence upon the function of the ventricular muscle and their absence is a marker of severe cardiac damage. On the other hand, *about half of the survivors of myocardial infarction have mild damage to the ventricle* and exercise testing in these patients will often show a physical capacity within the normal range and such patients should be able to enjoy normal, physically active lives. An important aspect of cardiac rehabilitation is the assessment of patients incapacity in these terms, so as to be able to offer a prognosis as regards functional recovery and to initiate treatment where it is called for.

Coronary artery disease

A myocardial infarct nearly always implies that a major coronary artery or one of its larger branches has been occluded. Patients will differ considerably in the extent of atheroma that is present in the remaining vessels, and this will determine whether they suffer from angina. It is also a powerful risk factor influencing expectation of life. *The 'gold standard' for the assessment of coronary disease during life is the coronary angiogram,* and some would recommend coronary angiography in every patient surviving a myocardial infarct. However, resources are insufficient to provide such a service and there is good evidence that patients with severe residual disease can be identified with a high degree of accuracy by the use of less expensive and non-invasive exercise tests.

In the past, the prevalence of angina after myocardial infarction was frequently underestimated. Occasionally, angina is improved by myocardial infarction if a small area of ischaemic muscle is converted into scar tissue. More often, angina is present after myocardial infarction and an important clinical clue to the presence of residual disease in the remaining coronary vessels. When the patient is seen in the early convalescent phase he may be undertaking very little in the way of physical exertion and so may not stress himself enough in order to reveal angina. In the past, patients were often advised to avoid any activity, and this advice would tend to conceal this complication. Exercise testing, therefore plays an important part in bringing to light severe residual disease after myocardial infarction.

Progression of disease

For the first year or two after a myocardial infarct, the prognosis can be gauged with considerable accuracy by assessment of the degree of muscle damage and the residual coronary disease. However, in the longer term, prognosis will also be much influenced by whether or not the disease progresses.

Measures to halt progress of the disease are an aspect of secondary prevention and must be considered along with other rehabilitation techniques and incorporated with them.

The most important single step the patient can take to reduce the risk of progression is to stop smoking. The evidence that correction of lipid abnormalities will have a very marked effect following myocardial infarction is slender, but nevertheless it seems a reasonable objective and it is certainly relevant if the patient undergoes coronary artery bypass grafting in order to

---

Secondary prevention
- Stop smoking
- Reduce a high cholesterol
- Increase exercise
- ? Alter personality

---

try and prevent the development of atheroma in the grafts. The role of exercise and secondary prevention will be considered later, but the evidence suggests that it has some benefit. The question of whether alteration of personality traits is practicable and would have a significant effect on prognosis remains unresolved at the present time.

Effects of bed rest and inactivity

The prolonged bed rest and reduced activity formerly advised in myocardial infarction have already been alluded to. The deleterious cardiovascular effects of enforced rest have been studied extensively together with the beneficial effects of exercise and training[4]. It has generally been assumed that some of the disability noted by patients, whose heart disease is mild, may be caused by enforced rest. In the past this may well have been so, but the current practice of much earlier mobilization and resumption of active life outside hospital must have reduced the deconditioning effect of rest during the acute phase[4]. The enforced rest studied by physiologists in the classic experiments on physical training was usually of the order of six weeks absolute bed rest for the treatment of a severe fracture, but few patients with infarction are now rested as long or completely as this.

Recent studies have suggested that mild cases of myocardial infarction, without angina and treated with modern regimes, have normal exercise tolerance[5]. Nowadays there seems little need for physical training as a routine measure to counteract the inactivity of the acute phase. However, physical training may still be beneficial as a measure of hastening resumption of activity and as a method of treatment of angina.

Psychological factors

Although all physical disease has psychological effects, myocardial infarction appears particularly serious in this respect, and anxiety and depression have been noted frequently. They are sometimes more disabling than the physical disease and there appears to be little or no correlation between the extent of the physical incapacity and the severity of the psychological disturbance. Since the effects of physical and psychological factors are additive, the recovery is likely to be particularly slow in patients with both, while patients who are free of unnecessary anxiety may be able to cope remarkably well with severe physical disability.

A few patients may require specialized psychiatric treatment and many more benefit from simple advice, explanation and support. Physical training is often accompanied by a marked improvement in morale, which is of considerable clinical benefit, even though the mechanism by which it occurs remains uncertain.

Social factors

Doctors differ in their opinion of how far they should involve themselves in the social consequence of disease but, in the case of myocardial infarction, there can be no doubt that complete recovery may be hindered or prevented altogether by such factors. This is particularly obvious when return to work is considered as an index of successful rehabilitation. The combination of a conservative approach to medical treatment with a national social security system, which removes the financial burden of sickness, will encourage prolonged inactivity. Inevitably some patients find themselves unable to undertake their original work, either because of physical incapacity or for legal reasons. What happens then will be determined largely by non-medical social factors. A large firm may offer alternative work but a small one may be unable to do so. In the latter case, the patient may become unemployed in one country but in another he may be classified as retired and given a permanent pension. In both cases, he may be perfectly capable of work if the right kind could be found. Clearly the doctor's power to help in such cases may be very limited. He can and should give authoritative advice to employers about his patient's capacity for work based on his knowledge of the acute illness and assessment by clinical evaluation and exercise testing. His representations on the patient's behalf may make all the difference between an active happy life and a restricted, boring and sad one.

Exercise tests and training

Exercise testing

The exercise test plays an important part in a rehabilitation programme and it also illustrates the physiology of exercise and the effects of physical training. The details of the exercise protocol may vary according to the equipment available and the local custom, but the principles remain similar for all such tests.

The test aims to study the effects of exercise up to the maximum that the patient can achieve. Since this is unknown before the test, exercise commences at a low, easy, level of work and gradually increases during the test to the patient's maximum – or to some pre-determined submaximal level. While sub-maximal testing may be preferable in some circumstances, such as a pre-discharge test soon after a myocardial infarct, a maximum test is more informative and safe when supervised by experienced staff. At each level of work

---

Measurement during exercise test
- heart rate
- Blood pressure
- ECG change – ST depression
  arrhythmias

---

during the test, measurements are made of heart rate and blood pressure. These determine the heart's requirements for oxygen and are therefore important in coronary disease. The ECG is used to record the heart rate and any arrhythmias and to detect depression of the ST segment as an index of myocardial ischaemia. The changes during a typical test are shown in Figure 3.1.

The exercise can be performed either on a *motor-driven treadmill* or on a *stationary cycle ergometer*. Each method has its own advantages but, overall, there is little to choose between them. On a cycle ergometer, the work level is measured directly in watts. On the treadmill, different levels of work are set by various combinations of speed and gradient, which are standardized in a number of protocols – the 'Bruce protocol' is the one in widest use.

Figure 3.1 shows approximate equivalent levels of work for both systems of measurement with some ordinary levels of activity for comparison. Exercise tests using treadmills or cycle ergometers have almost completely replaced methods using steps or simple walking. The more modern tests enable the level of work to be measured accurately and to be reproduced exactly on subsequent tests, thus making it possible to measure changes over time. The fact that the patient is stationary

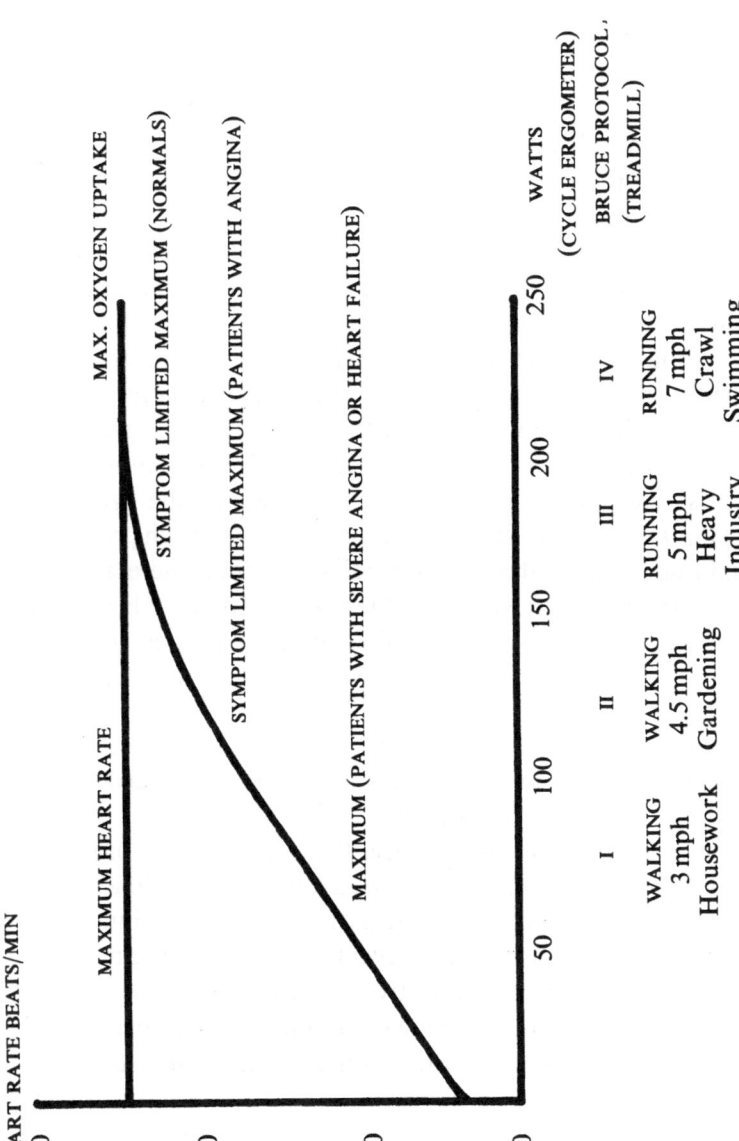

Figure 3.1 Approximate levels of work on cycle ergometer and treadmill

while exercising makes it much easier to monitor ECG during exercise. It should be borne in mind that a properly conducted exercise test is quite expensive and requires at least two staff for about half an hour.

Some confusion arises because of the different 'maximum' points at which the test may be terminated and which are illustrated in the figure. The maximum oxygen uptake (or aerobic power) defines the maximum capacity of the circulation to transport oxygen and the maximum capacity for continuous exercise. In clinical medicine, few patients can be persuaded to exert themselves to this level and more practical, lower, maximal levels are used. Heart rate rises linearly with work load to a maximum heart rate, which is constant for each individual, though falling with increasing age. An exercise test may be continued until the individual's maximum heart rate is reached, or it may be terminated at the *predicted* maximum heart rate based on the patient's age. Such predicted maximum heart rates are less reliable, since there is considerable individual variation amounting to ±20 beats per minute around the average value for a given age. Finally, submaximal exercise tests often proceed to a pre-determined 'target' heart rate, which is usually 85% of the predicted average maximum heart rate for the patient's age. Such calculations suffer from the inaccuracy already mentioned for all predicted maximum heart rates.

For patients with heart disease, the best and most practical maximum is the *symptom limited* maximum work load. This is the level of work at which the patient cannot continue. The nature of the symptom that prevents him continuing must be stated. This endpoint is subjective, especially when the patient stops because of geneal fatigue or simple lack of effort. When angina is the limiting symptom, on the other hand, the endpoint proves to be very reliable and reproducible on successive tests. The response of heart rate and blood pressure to exercise is altered by various drugs, particularly beta-blockers – they lower both variables at each level of exertion and also reduce the maximum heart rate.

HEART RATE BEATS/MIN

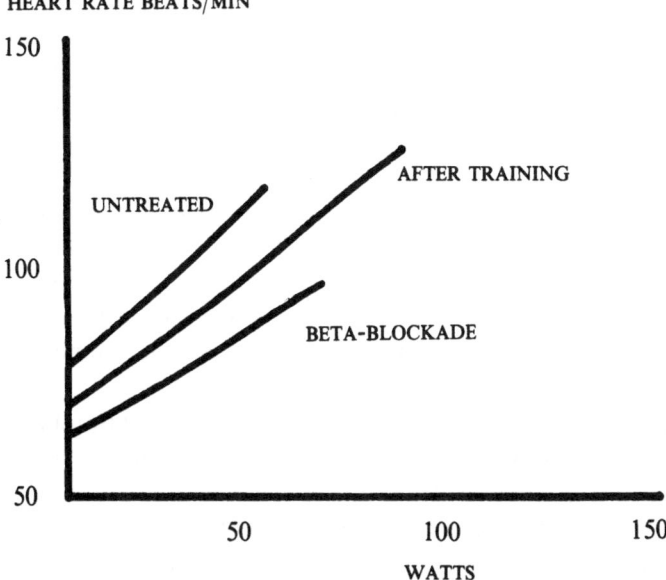

Figure 3.2 Heart rate response and exercise capacity in a patient with angina: untreated; after exercise training; and, for comparison, under treatment with beta-blocking drugs

Exercise training

Physical training reduces heart rate at each level of submaximal exercise, but has little effect on maximum heart rate, therefore the trained subject can attain higher levels of maximum work (Fig. 3.2). In patients with coronary disease, the most beneficial aspect of the training effect is the reduction in submaximal levels of heart rate and blood pressure. Because the demands of the heart for oxygen are largely determined by these variables, this means that the heart requires less oxygen for a given level of work and angina is less likely to occur. Physical training that is sufficient to produce this effect is most beneficial among those patients who are limited by angina and the effect on heart rate and blood pressure is the most important mechanism.

A number of studies have attempted to see if physical training has a beneficial effect on the heart itself and if higher oxygen demands from the heart muscle can be met[6]. The evidence suggests that some improvement in oxygen supply to the myocardium may well occur, but it remains true that the greatest part of the improvement is likely to result from a reduction in oxygen demand due to the change in heart rate and blood pressure. The beneficial effects of training on the circulation are to some extent specific to the kind of exercise performed during the training programme. Training using the arms affects the response to arm exercise more than to leg exercise and vice versa. A practical training programme should therefore include a wide range of exercise.

It is necessary to correct the widely held misapprehension that cardiac rehabilitation is no more than the provision of facilities for physical training. Nevertheless, a training programme is one of the most distinctive features of rehabilitation and usually forms part of a rehabilitation service.

Effective physical training is capable of producing measureable and beneficial changes in the circulation but hard exercise, sufficient to raise the heart rate to about 140 beats per minute is required to do it. It is a mistake to consider that all the benefits of training are dependent upon these specific physiological effects. Lighter training, which is insufficient to cause physiological changes, may be of great value in the management of patients and is considerably easier and cheaper to provide – as well as being acceptable and popular with many patients, who would have doubts about a more vigorous programme and might well refuse to attend or drop out during

---

Benefits of exercise class
- Reduces myocardial O_2 demand
- Improves agility
- Boosts confidence
- Observation of patient's progress
- Improves doctor/patient rapport

the course. The benefits of light training are summarized in Figure 3.2. It is often assumed that where no measurable training effect on the circulation can be shown, the benefits must be entirely psychological. This seems an over simple view. The improvement in posture, agility, vigour and confidence may not be measureable but is commented upon by all observers and may be compared with the improvement that one sees after an active and energetic holiday. The regular exercise classes also offer an admirable opportunity to observe the progress of patients during convalescence, which is particularly useful where symptoms are difficult to interpret or where spontaneous improvement is expected. In this respect it supplements the information obtained during the exercise test in a way, which is scientifically less precise and reproduceable but is often – more realistic, closer to the exercise the patient will take in everyday life and repeatable twice a week at little cost. Finally, the exercise class provides a regular opportunity for contact and discussion between patient and doctor in a uniquely informal setting, quite different from the clinic.

For these reasons, a doctor should always be present at the exercise sessions, not only for reasons of safety, but also to take advantage of the opportunities the classes provide for good clinical medicine.

Exercise programme

The exact format of the exercise programme will vary according to the facilities available. Patients can be taught to exercise themselves at home following an exercise test and with regular contact and supervision, but an exercise class at the hospital remains the cheapest and most effective method in most circumstances. Exercise is more effective the more often it is undertaken, but a class two or three times a week is practical. A doctor and physiotherapist can supervise a class of 10 or 12 patients.

The most convenient method of organizing the class is to

have the patients perform circuit training, in which they follow a circuit of some 10 exercises for a period of about 5 to 10 minutes followed by 5 minutes rest. Four such circuits can be included in a typical hour's session. Some control is desirable over the degree of effort that each patient is making. Some centres use radio telemetry of the ECG but simpler methods will suffice. We measure the patient's pulse rate before and immediately after each circuit and the time taken is noted from an individual stop clock.

When patients first attend the class, the circuit is unfamiliar to them and the time taken is inevitably slow. Patients are usually limited to two or three circuits during these early visits. As the circuits are learned, the speed automatically increases and the patients gradually increase their effort to match that of others in the class. Only occasionally is it necessary to urge someone to work harder or to take it a bit easier.

Some patients will develop symptoms during the classes and these must be evaluated and treated appropriately. Medication may be altered and the effects can be observed in subsequent visits to the class. Sometimes, it will become apparent that angina or breathlessness is more severe than was anticipated and speedy referral for coronary angiography will be the appropriate response. In order to obtain the greatest value from the exercise programme, it is highly desirable that the medical staff running it should be in clinical charge of the patient and able to make these alterations to treatment without delay.

The light exercise programme forms an excellent introduction for the new patient. When patients are allowed to set their own pace in this way they usually develop heart rates of around 120 beats per minute after each circuit. This is insufficient to produce a physiological training effect within a few weeks. To achieve such an effect, harder exertion is required sufficient to raise the heart to around 140 beats per minute. In our experience, patients will not usually exercise to this level without additional stimulus and control during the class. Circuits can be supplemented by exercise on a cycle ergometer to levels of work sufficient to achieve these higher heart rates. The work loads necessary for this can be calculated from the results of the exercise test which should always be done before hard training of this kind.

An exercise programme is a most valuable adjunct to the systematic follow-up of the convalescent coronary patient. A simple programme of light exercise can be undertaken by nearly all patients including those with moderate heart failure or angina and is popular with the patients and greatly appreciated by them. Harder exercise, sufficient to produce the training effects already described, is probably unnecessary for the majority of patients but may be of benefit to some. These will include patients with intractable angina and patients who need or desire to increase their exercise capacity. Such patients might include those who have suffered deconditioning from prolonged immobility or who wish to take up new activities. For these selected patients, a 'second level' programme with harder exercise for a longer time would be ideal. If facilities do not exist for this they can be accommodated in the general class.

SELLY OAK REHABILITATION SCHEME

The scheme of cardiac rehabilitation shown in Table 3.1 is one that has evolved at Selly Oak Hospital over a period of 15 years and that attempts to implement these principles in a practical and economical way. It uses simple methods and a minimum of staff. Medical care is provided by the same medical team throughout and we aim to include patients with all grades of severity of disease.

In accordance with good general principles of rehabilitation, the process starts in the coronary care unit during the first days of the illness. At this time, the diagnosis is established by serial ECG's and enzyme measurements. If angina without infarction is suspected, an attempt is made to obtain ECG records during attacks of pain and arrangements may be made

Table 3.1 The coronary follow-up clinic

Recent diagnosis	Infarct? severe angina? other?
Complications	Heart failure, reinfarction, embolus, etc.
Present treatment	Still needed?
Job	Demands physical and mental, driving, legal?
Present activity	How much, how often, how fast?
Symptoms	Angina, breathlessness, palpitations, etc.
Lipids	Measured on admission or before illness
Previous hypertension	BP level, complications
Tobacco	Should have stopped
Physical examination	Rhythm, heart size, gallops, crepitations
Blood pressure	
ECG	Compared with record in hospital
Chest X-ray	Heart size, lungs for LV failure
Action	Advice
	Wife
	Exercise test
	Physical training
	Job, employer
	Letters, GP, employer, etc.
	Dietary advice
Progress in gym or at follow-up	
Return to work	
Follow-up at work	
Discharge	

for pre-discharge exercise testing a few days later. Where infarction has occurred, daily assessments are made for evidence of heart failure, clinical signs of gallop rhythm, abnormal cardiac pulsation and rales in the chest. The chest X-ray is examined for enlargement of the heart and left ventricular failure.

The coronary care unit has proved to be outstandingly successful in stopping patients smoking and few fail to give it up, at least in the short term. Blood is taken for a fasting lipid profile on the first morning after admission, when it is a fair

Assessment in CCU
- Gallop rhyythm
- Pulmonary crepitations
- Abnormal cardiac pulsation
- Chest X-ray for – cardiac enlargement
  pulmonary congestion

estimate of the pre-morbid lipid levels can act as a guide to the need for treatment later. If this opportunity on the first day is missed, lipid levels measured later are reduced by the metabolic effects of the illness and give a misleading impression of the chronic state.

Patients with definite infarction or severe angina who are 65 years old or less have their notes marked while in the CCU, so that an appointment will be made for the coronary follow-up clinic approximately four weeks after admission. Patients are admitted under the physician of the day and care on the CCU is shared with the cardiologist. Patients seen at the coronary follow-up clinic are cared for by the cardiologists thereafter.

The coronary follow-up clinic was the first element of the rehabilitation service to be established and remains the focal point of the scheme. Its principal purposes are assessment and advice (Table 3.2).

Table 3.2 Characteristics of the clinic

Organized follow-up of all cases

Assessment of the effects of the disease in functional terms

Definition of the patient's objectives and hopes

Discussion of fears and worries

Discussion with family

Communication with other doctors, workplace etc.

Establishment of a plan for convalescence.

The information gathered during the acute illness is reviewed in order to assess the certainty of the diagnosis and the severity of the damage to the heart that has occurred. Complications are noted and their significance is assessed. *For those in work, resumption of employment is the biggest single milestone on the path to recovery and one of the main objectives of the service.* For all patients, we try to discover something of their way of life and their needs and objectives. Unfortunately, many are unemployed at the present time and this removes one of the strongest spurs to recovery. It is important to motivate such people to achieve the best recovery possible and to enjoy life.

We ask what physical activity the patient is undertaking at the present time and what symptoms have been found. Most at this stage are doing very little and are often symptom free. Sometimes this gives a misleading by favourable impression of their exercise capacity, which will be exposed later during the exercise test. Nevertheless, the patient's present level of activity makes the best starting point for advice about future activity and exercise.

Examination of the heart, the ECG and the chest X-ray complete the assessment and supplement the information obtained during the acute illness.

By now a reasonably complete picture should be available and the patient should have this assessment explained with the wife or husband present, so that both hear the identical form of words. The same assessment should be conveyed to the general practitioner and he should be kept informed of every subsequent development until the patient is eventually returned to his sole care.

Wives will often show particular concern about diet. While evidence for the benefit of dietary modification after infarction is uncertain, such a request for information should be met. Dietary advice can be a useful public health measure for the family and people are particularly receptive at this time.

Advice is given about increasing exercise from the present level with an indication of the rate of progress which can be expected. For the typical patient we usually tell them to aim at a gradual progressive resumption of all normal everyday activities over the course of the next four weeks, so that a return to work could be contemplated two or three months after admission. This advice must be individualized, taking into account the patient's physical capacity both before and after the illness, the inclination for exercise he has shown so far and the levels he requires in the future. Other questions will arise at this stage. While exercise and work may be the preoccupations of the doctor, driving and sex are likely to be of greater concern to the patient. Both activities can be resumed once the patient is doing other ordinary light everyday activities – such as walking half a mile, going to the shops and doing jobs around the house.

For most patients, the final step at the follow-up clinic is to arrange an exercise test a day or two later.

Even if no facilities exist for exercise testing or supervised exercise, a clinic organized along these lines can achieve most of the objectives of rehabilitation. The characteristics of the clinic are summarized in Table 3.2 and represent the principles of good rehabilitation. We have found that such a clinic (on its own) will reduce unnecessary invalidism, improve return to work and identify patients who require further investigation. The most important single addition to the clinic alone is the exercise test, which is arranged a few days after the clinic visit.

All of the benefit of the clinic may be lost if the assessment, information and plans made are not transmitted to those who need to know them. Foremost among these are the *general practitioner,* but great help can also be achieved by writing to the *works medical officer* or to the *personnel officer.* In my experience, firms will do much to help their employees if they are informed and asked to. On the other hand, once a decision has been taken to dismiss an employee, it can seldom be reversed.

Nearly all patients undergo a symptom limited maximum exercise test. The small number too ill to undertake such a test are shown to be high risk cases who should be immediately considered for further invasive investigation by coronary angiography. Occasionally we have dispensed with the formal test in a patient who has few symptoms and who is coming to the exercise classes, but we have often regretted the omission and had to arrange a test later. Symptoms often arise in the exercise class which are difficult to interpet and which can be better understood after a formal test.

We usually start the test at 20 watts and increase the load every minute by 10 or 20 watts according to the patients response. We are particularly interested in the maximum tolerated work load and the symptoms that limit it. In the absence of drugs that influence heart rate, the heart rate at a standard load (such as 100 watts) is a guide to the stroke volume and function of the left ventricle. For this reason we prefer to avoid the use of beta blocking drugs before the test, unless there is a particular indication. Alternatively, the drugs may be withdrawn for a few days before the test, though this may result in an exacerbation of angina. Patients unable to achieve a level of 50 watts will be unable to undertake normal activities and are referred for investigation. Patients who can exceed 120 watts can usually work and will be able to manage the exercise class. Between these two levels are patients limited to something between 50 and 100 watts who need careful observation. We usually bring them to the exercise class for training and supervision. Frequently, their medication will be adjusted in the class and in some cases they will prove to be severely disabled and will require investigation. Others will improve over the next few weeks and will eventually be discharged on medical treatment.

Most patients join the exercise classes which are held twice a week and last an hour. After a preliminary relaxation period, patients undertake a circuit of 12 exercises in their own time. Each circuit takes about eight minutes for the newer and less fit patients, and about four minutes for the most active and those about to leave the class. To this basic routine can be added exercise on a cycle ergometer (based on the exercise test) to raise the heart rate to 140 beats per minute, or weight training to improve the strength and endurance of those who will return to physically demanding work.

Patients usually attend the class for a period of four to eight weeks and are then discharged to work or to their own devices. Arrangements are always made to see them in the clinic some weeks after return to work in order to ensure that no unforeseen difficulties have arisen.

OTHER FORMS OF HEART DISEASE

Other forms of heart disease can benefit from physical training. Patients with angina and patients who have recently undergone coronary surgery or valve replacement may well be more deconditioned than many after a myocardial infarct. The fact that surgical patients often come from a very wide

---

Useful practical points

- The aims of coronary rehabilitation are physical recovery, psychological acceptance of the condition and a return to normal living
- The most important factor in preventing recurrence of a heart attack is to give up smoking
- Exercise testing is the best method of screening for post-coronary patients who may need coronary artery surgery
- Exercise training is useful after a heart attack to improve cardiac performance and reduce myocardial oxygen requirements
- Liaison between the specialist and the general practitioner, as well as the works medical officer or personnel officer, is of considerable value in getting the patient back to work after the heart attack

geographical area makes this kind of structured programme more difficult to implement. Physical training is often useful for patients awaiting coronary surgery and appears to lead to faster and more complete recovery provided the patient is able to take part.

SUMMARY

The objectives of Cardiac Rehabilitation should be the concern of all doctors and much can be achieved by simple methods, if the will and interest are there. In the hospital setting, a structured rehabilitation programme can be provided at relatively low cost. The patients are still passing through a phase of their disease in which medical supervision and assessment is important and the programme needs to be under the care of a physician. In my view, he should be in clinical care of the patients while they remain in the rehabilitation programme, so that treatment can be altered and planned with the minimum of delay and the best use made of the unparalleled opportunities for observation at first hand of the patient's progress.

REFERENCES

1. World Health Organisation (1983). *Rehabilitation and comprehensive secondary prevention after acute myocardial infarction.* (Copenhagen: World Health Organisation)
2. Nagle R., Gangola R. and Picton-Robinson, I. (1971). Factors influencing return to work after myocardial infarction. *Lancet,* **2,** 454
3. DeBusk, R.F., Houston, N., Haskell, W., Fry, G. and Parker, M. (1979). Exercise training soon after myocardial infarction. *Am. J. Cardiol.,* **44,** 1223
4. Saltin, B., Blomquist, G., Mitchell, J.H., Johnson, R.L., Wildenthal, K. and Chapman, C.B. (1968). Response to sub-maximal and maximal exercise after bed rest and training. *Circ.,* **38,** Suppl. 7
5. Borer, J.S., Rosing, D.R., Miller, R.H. *et al.* (1980). Natural history

of left ventricular function during one year after acute myocardial infarction. *Am. J. Cardiol.*, **46,** 1–12

6. Sanne, H. (1973). Exercise tolerance and physical training of non-selected patients after myocardial infarction. *Acta Med. Scand.*, Suppl. 551

4

THE MANAGEMENT OF ANGINA

G. Jackson

INTRODUCTION

There are many causes of chest pain. The principal diagnostic problem is separating cardiac pain from muscular, oesophageal or functional pain, perhaps secondary to the hyperventilation syndrome (Table 4.1).

Angina is a clinical diagnosis based on the doctor's interpretation of a set of symptoms. The diagnosis of angina is aided by the electrocardiogram but it is most important to realize that a normal resting ECG does not rule out significant coronary artery disease.

Angina is not a diagnosis to be made lightly, nor a diagnosis to persevere with if there are reasonable doubts. It is all very well to outline the classical presentation and some of the pitfalls but in the real world a significant minority have a chest pain symptom complex, which is impossible to pin down. These people should always be evaluated further for the diagnosis of angina may have major social and family implications – jobs may be threatened, manhood or womanhood challenged and fear of sudden death or a heart attack preoccupy the family unit.

Table 4.1   Some differential features of chest pain

Angina	—See Table 4.3.
Oesophageal	—Not exertional. Rarely radiates to left arm. Worse when lying flat or after a large meal. Relieved by belching, standing, antacids *but* also by GTN and Nifedipine.
Pericarditis	—Sharp pain worse on inspiration and lying flat. Relieved by shallow breathing and standing. Often pyrexial. Rub may be audible.
Pulmonary	—Pleuritic pain, worse with breathing, often localized. Frequent cough or haemoptysis. Rub audible.
Musculoskeletal	—Positional, localized, reproduced by pressure. Sharp, suddenly severe. May be tightness due to pectoral spasm. May be deep to breast in female.
Functional	—Hyperventilation. Patient easily breathless, frequent sighs, anxious, often young female. Musculoskeletal pain may be associated.
Mitral valve prolapse	—Mostly atypical but some typical pains commoner in younger women who may also hyperventilate. Frequently pain *after* exercise when fatigued.

TYPES OF ANGINA

1. Stable angina

It was William Heberden (1710–1801) who introduced the term 'angina pectoris' and there is little room for improvement in his classical description of its clinical effects[1].

'There is a disorder of the breast, marked with strong and peculiar symptoms, considerable for the kind of danger belonging to it, and not extremely rare, of which I do not recollect any mention among medical authors. The seat of it, and sense of strangling and anxiety with which it is attended, may make it not improperly be called Angina pectoris.

Those who are afflicted with it, are seized while they are walking, and more particularly when they walk soon after eating, with a painful and most disagreeable sensation in the breast, which seems as if it would take their life away, if it were to increase or to continue: the moment they stand still, all this uneasiness vanishes. In all other respects the patients are at the beginning of this disorder perfectly well, and in particular have no shortness of breath, from which it is totally different.'

He did not, however, differentiate angina pectoris from cardiac infarction, nor did he divide it into stable or unstable forms – yet so precise were his observations that unwittingly he records these variations.

'After it has continued some months, it will not cease so instantaneously upon standing still; and it will come on, not only when the persons are walking but when they are lying down and oblige them to rise up out of their beds every night for many months . . . '

The nature of the pain

Ischaemic pain should be defined from the following questions:

(1) Site — Whereabouts in the chest is the pain?

(2) Radiation — Does it go anywhere else besides the chest?

(3) Character — What does it feel like?

(4) Cause—What brings the pain on?

(5) Relief—What do you do when you have the pain – what makes it go away?

Site

This is usually retrosternal. The patient signals the squeezing constricting feeling by clenching his fist over the sternum (Fig.

4.1). The patient may identify the location by moving the flat of his hand across the chest but he does *not* point to the pain.

Radiation

The pain may spread to the back or throat giving a choking sensation, or involve the jaw simulating toothache. Frequently the pain radiates to the left arm, less commonly to the right, and often to both arms. Cardiac pain usually travels under the axilla whereas muscular pain is usually experienced over the shoulder or outside the upper arm (Fig. 4.2).

Pain in the back may lead the patient to believe it is muscular or 'arthritis' and pain in the epigastrium 'indigestion'. The most dangerous presentation is of pain in the referral sites only. This can lead to visits to rheumatologists or gastro-enterologists. Thankfully, an exertional or emotional component usually clarifies the diagnosis, but from time to time patients will present with such a mixture of symptoms that it is impossible to be sure on history alone. The most common sites of chest pain are shown in Table 4.2[2].

Character

The pain is usually a tightness – not severe, more of an ache – a heaviness, a constriction, or very frequently a sensation of breathlessness (tightness). Those who experience angina as breathlessness should be asked, 'What do you mean by breath-lessness? Do you feel tight in the chest or are you panting for breath?' Too many people are on bronchodilators or diuretics when they should be on antianginal therapy. The mildness of the pain and sometimes its relationship to a heavy meal make it easily misdiagnosed by the patient as indigestion. Severe pain, which is sharp is rarely cardiac, is usually muscular and can be pointed to by the patient – i.e. it is localized rather than the generalized nature of cardiac pain. The clenched fist sign is helpful but one of the features of cardiac pain is a difficulty

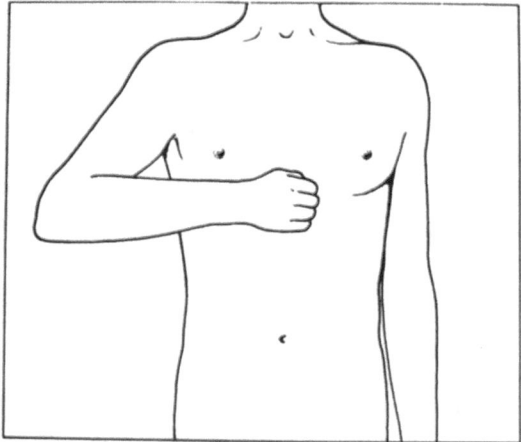

Figure 4.1   Clenched fist sign with the patient clearly identifying the location and character of the pain

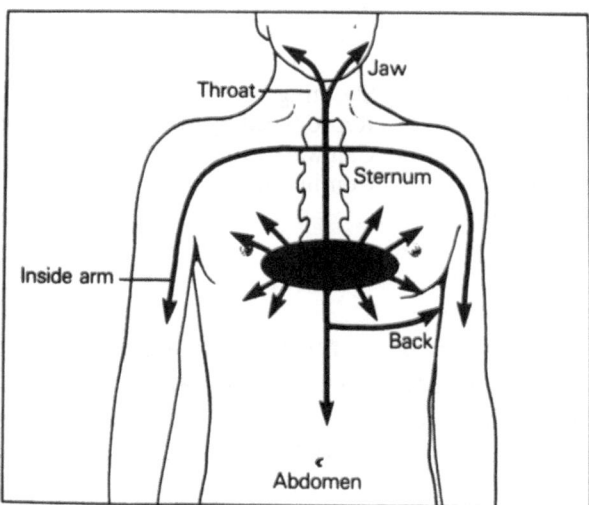

Figure 4.2   Site and radiation of cardiac pain

Table 4.2　Site of anginal pain in 150 successive ambulatory patients[2]

Location of pain	% Sole involvement	% Involvement at any time
Anterior chest	34.0	96.0
Left arm (upper)	0.7	30.7
Left arm (lower)	1.3	29.3
Right arm (upper)	0	10.0
Right arm (lower)	0	13.3
Back	0.7	16.7
Epigastrium	0.7	3.3
Forehead	0	6.0
Neck	2.0	22.0
Chin and perioral area	0	8.7

Table 4.3　Characteristics of chest pain

Cardiac	Non-cardiac
Tightness	Sharp (not severe)
Pressure	Knife-like
Weight	Stabbing
Constriction	'Like a stitch'
Ache	'Like needle'
Dull	Pricking feeling
Squeezing feeling	Shooting
Soreness	Reproduced by pressure or position
Crushing	Can walk around with it
'Like a band'	Continuous: 'It's there all day, Doc'
Breathless (tightness)	

the patient has in being precise – its almost as though the mildness puts him off. Whilst in Table 4.3 most of the features are summarized local dialects are important – in South London, for example, 'sharp' means 'severe' not 'knife-like'.

Causes

The commonest cause of angina is obstructive coronary artery disease. When the arteries are narrowed by over 70%, blood supply is reduced[3]. The coronary arteries fill in diastole, so the more rapid the rate the greater the demand and the less time for coronary filling.

We have a classical supply and demand problem. Any factor that increases heart rate may induce pain if the balance is upset. Pain usually predictably follows exertion, temperature

> Causes of angina
> - Heart rate ↑
> - Exertion
> - Temperature ↓ ↑
> - Hot bath
> - Large meal
> - Emotion

change, a hot bath, or a large meal. The importance here is of the predictable nature of the pain. Day-to-day variations occur, perhaps secondary to cold or windy weather or exercising too soon after a meal. Emotion frequently induces pain from the extremes of fright and anger to exciting television or vivid dreams. Patients who wake up with pain at night may not be unstable (see later) but have heart rate induced angina secondary to dreaming.

Pain relief

Slowing the heart rate, reducing the workload (demand) on the heart by standing still, or reducing the pace of activity will relieve the pain. Patients gaze into shop windows, sit on benches or use their glyceryl trinitrate medication. Pain relief is rapid, invariably less than five minutes, which means that antacids will help because the patient has to stand still to use them – the indigestion fallacy being reinforced in his mind.

2. Unstable angina

This condition has many names, the most common being crescendo angina, pre-infarction syndrome, the intermediate coronary syndrome and acute coronary insufficiency.

Unstable angina is new or rapidly worsening pain or pain

> **Pain in unstable angina**
> - Recent
> - New
> - At rest
> - Persistent

at rest. The pain may be rapidly increasing in severity, more prolonged more frequent and superimposed on a previous stable background. New onset angina (within the first month) and rest pain signal this most dangerous condition.

3. Variant angina

This is also known as Prinzmetal's angina[4]. It is caused by spasm either superimposed on a fixed coronary lesion or in the presence of normal coronary arteries. It may rarely be exertional, but usually occurs at rest or in response to cold (Fig. 4.3). In some it has a consistent time in the day when it occurs, usually at night. The presence of ST elevation during the ischaemia separates it from the more usual ST depression of the other forms of angina. It is promptly relieved by nitrates and calcium antagonists, which reverse the vasospastic aetiology.

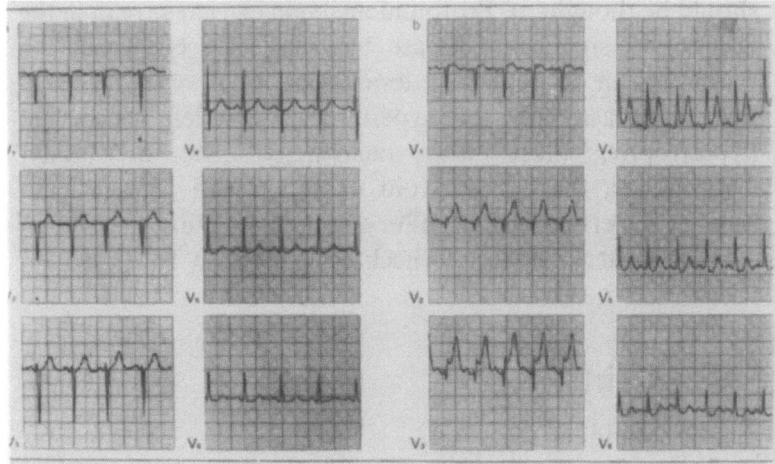

Figure 4.3 ST elevation of variant angina

AETIOLOGY

Obstructive coronary artery disease is the commonest cause of angina pectoris. Other conditions with or without co-existent coronary artery disease should be considered in the diagnosis. In the older patient, aortic stenosis and/or incompetence

Table 4.4 Aetiology of angina

(1)	Obstructive coronary artery disease
(2)	Coronary spasm (usually rest pain)
(3)	Aortic stenosis
(4)	Aortic incompetence
(5)	Left ventricular hypertrophy (hypertension, cardiomyopathy)
(6)	Anaemia
(7)	Thyrotoxicosis
(8)	Rapid or slow arrhythmias
(9)	Severe mitral stenosis
(10)	Primary pulmonary hypertension

should be thought of. Profound anaemia can cause pain in the absence of significant disease but may also bring out the symptoms in those whose lesions are mild or moderately severe. Occasionally the hypertensive with left ventricular hypertrophy, those with tachyarrhythmias or brady-arrhythmias, the hyperthyroid or those with primary pulmonary hypertension can suffer anginal pain independently of coronary artery disease. A check list is given in Table 4.4.

ASSESSMENT

1. Stable angina

Examination

This is invariably normal. When inspecting the patient ana-emia should be looked for. Signs of hyperlipidaemia include xanthomas on the hands, elbows, knees and ankles. Xan-thelasma (the eyelids) is surprisingly non-specific for hyper-lipidaemia, as is arcus senilis in those over 40 years of age. A younger person with an arcus is worthy of more detailed assessment.

The most frequent ausculatory finding is a 4th heart sound reflecting reduced ventricular compliance. Aortic stenosis and incompetence need excluding and a late systolic mitral murmur may represent ischaemia of the papillary muscles. Extra-systoles may occur with or without pain and a dyskinetic ventricle may be palpable. This may reflect old damage or ischaemia if present only during pain. The blood pressure may be elevated and signs of associated carotid or peripheral arterial disease should be sought.

Examination – NB Usually normal

Look for:

- Anaemia
- Hyperlipidaemic signs – Xanthomas
                                           Arcus senilis if below 40
                                           years of age

Ausculatory signs:

- 4th heart sound
- Aortic stenosis and incompetence
- Extra systoles
- Palpable dyskinetic ventricle
- Increased BP and associated corotid or peripheral
  arterial disease

Investigations

These questions need answering:

    (1) Who is at risk?

    (2) How do we identify them?

    (3) Can we modify the risk?

The patient with severe symptoms, in spite of medical therapy, has selected himself for further investigation. Here our decision is simple. Our major problem is correlating mild symptoms with extent of disease. Unfortunately those with severe life threatening disease may have minimal symptoms on medical therapy.

Who is at risk?

The European Coronary Surgery Study[5] showed that surgery improved the quantity and quality of life of those with mild to moderate symptoms, who had left main stem stenosis (Figs.

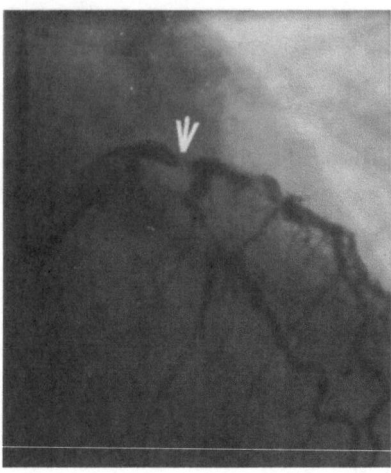

Figure 4.4   Left main stem disease (arrow). Additional distal disease also

4.4, 4.5), significant stenosis in all the major coronary arteries and two vessel disease, where one of the vessels involved was the left anterior descending before the first septal branch. Single vessel disease or other two vessel disease was not associated with an obvious surgical benefit – in other words, prognostically those patients should be managed on symptoms. This study clearly made the identification of patients with severe disease very important.

A subsequent study – the Coronary Artery Surgical Study (CASS)[6] – from America provided conflicting results. This study excluded left main disease and included only those with no or very minimal symptoms. The selection for entry to the study was odd in that only 780 out of 16 626 assessed were included. Considering the prevalence of coronary artery surgery in America and the number of institutions involved (15) this recruitment rate indicates an unusual and very highly selected group of people. Indeed the number of authors on the paper approached 400! The CASS study showed overall that medical therapy was no different from surgical therapy in terms of survival but that the surgical group experienced less subsequent angina[7]. Subsequent analysis identified groups who were more likely to benefit from surgery, in particular those with a reduced ejection fraction and those with an abnormal exercise test[8].

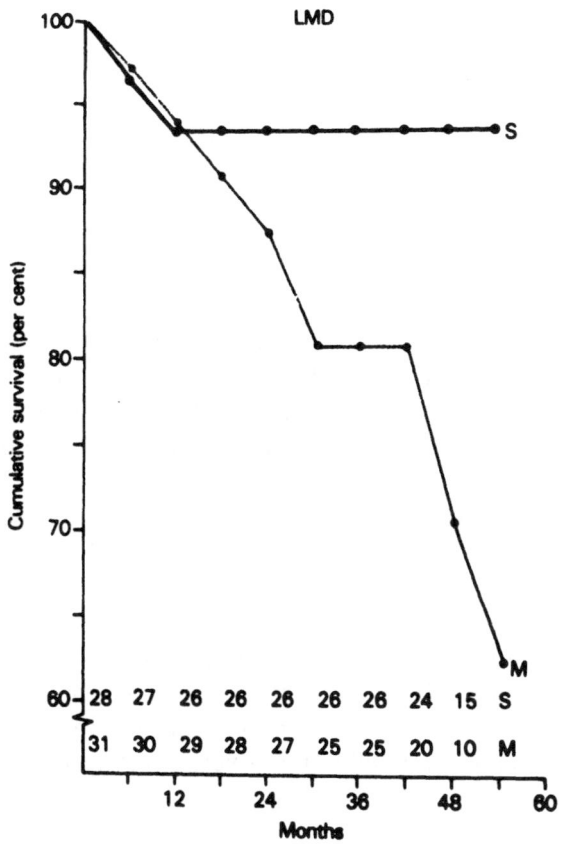

Figure 4.5 Improved five year survival after coronary bypass surgery in patients with left main disease (LMD): S = surgery; M = medical therapy

How can we rationalize the two studies?

Firstly there is no doubt that exercise testing is essential to exclude left main stem disease.

Secondly those with a positive exercise test need further evaluation by angiography.

Thirdly there is no need to rush into evaluating those with minimal symptoms but in due course an exercise ECG is desirable.

Identifying those at risk

General

Coronary angiography is the only absolute test. Those below 40 years of age should routinely undergo this procedure. We are making planning decisions for the next 20 to 30 years and therefore we need the maximum information to optimize management.

In patients over 40 years of age, treadmill exercise testing using a 12 lead ECG has proved very useful. The age limits I have chosen are arbitrary and rely on the accuracy of the treadmill ECG predicting those with or without coronary artery disease. There is no doubt that I would routinely investigate the under 50s if my waiting time was less. Thus, with our limited resources, I can reduce the number of routine angiograms and hopefully offer a better service to those with a definite need.

Specific

1. *Screening.* Screening the asymptomatic patient with resting and exercise electrocardiography is no longer recommended because of a high incidence (66%) of false positives[9]. However, in those with a strong familial incidence perhaps linked to an inherited hyperlipidaemia it makes sense to follow them more closely. Certainly the children and blood

relatives of a hyperlipidaemic coronary patient should be evaluated also.

2. *Exercise testing*. The treadmill exercise 12 lead ECG is a safe and accurate non-invasive test for the risk evaluation of

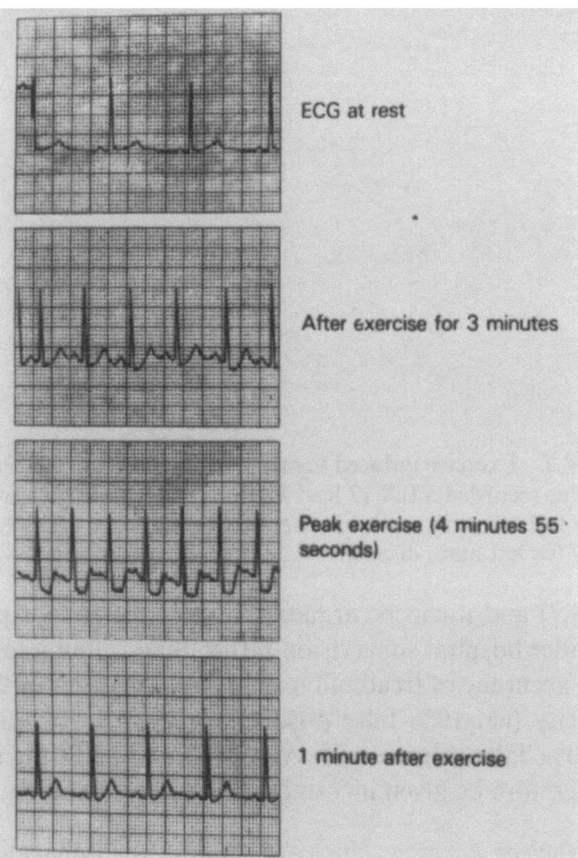

Figure 4.6   Exercise induced ST depression

patients with chest pain. The main endpoints are significant – ST segment depression of greater than 1 mm (Fig. 4.6), a slow recovery to normal, a fall in systolic blood pressure, angina at a low workload and dangerous arrhythmias such as ventricular tachycardia. Medical supervision is essential for though the risks are few, the consequences can be fatal[10]. The overall mortality is 1:10 000 tests and the non-fatal complication rate is 2.4:10 000[11]. The incidence of ventricular fibrillation is 1:5000

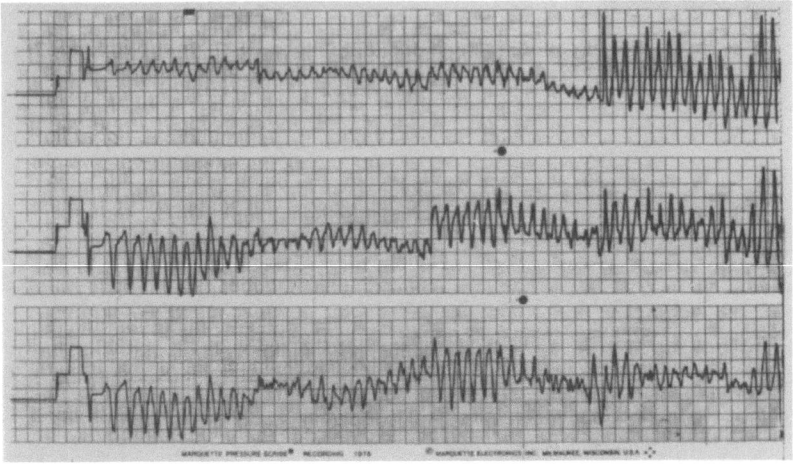

Figure 4.7   Exercise induced ventricular fibrillation. The ECG computer recorded a full 12 lead ECG as the patient collapsed. He made a full recovery and underwent successful emergency bypass surgery for left main disease

(Fig. 4.7) and it can be argued that it is better to experience this under hospital supervision rather than running for a bus.

The accuracy of treadmill testing is of the order of 90% for specificity (i.e. 10% false positives) and 80% for sensitivity (i.e. 20% false negatives)[11]. A small but significant number will therefore be given incorrect advice non-invasively.

3. *Nuclear imaging.* Nuclear scanning for ischaemia has a limited but helpful role in evaluation. It is useful when the resting ECG has characteristics which make it difficult to evaluate on exercise, particularly left bundle branch block.

It is also helpful when the patient cannot exercise for various reasons – such as arthritis, claudication or obstructive airways disease, or when the routine exercise ECG gives non-diagnostic or borderline information in a patient with an atypical story. Thallium-201 is taken up by perfused myocardium. Thus infarcted areas will be delineated and under exercise areas of reduced perfusion will be identified. This can be helpful regarding sensitivity, but appears no better than exercise testing on specificity[12].

Technetium-99 radionuclide left ventricular angiography is of great value in assessing left ventricular function[13]. Its role is probably related to risk assessment post infarction, though in those with angina and atypical features a clear indication of exercise induced ventricular dysfunction would precipitate the need for angiography.

At the present time in the angina patient 12 lead treadmill testing is the cheapest reliable non-invasive approach, with thallium imaging of use in important subsets or when reasonable doubts in diagnosis persist.

4. *Coronary angiography*. This is a specialist technique requiring a day in hospital. Though it is a quick (20–30 minutes) procedure with minimal risk (1:2000 death rate)[14], it is expensive. The approximate cost is £550 per procedure.

Under local anaesthetic, catheters are advanced either from the femoral artery (Judkins technique) or brachial artery (Sones technique). Contrast medium is injected into the coronary arteries in multiple views using hand injections and into the left ventricle under greater pressure via a pump. The patient experiences (besides fear) a warm sensation for 90 seconds after the left ventricular angiogram.

Coronary angiography accurately assesses the anatomy of the individual coronary arteries and their branches and the left ventriculogram identifies areas of dysfunction, which will influence management.

When asked who should undergo this procedure, the short and ideal answer is 'everyone with symptoms'. Given that left ventricular damage and the extent of coronary artery disease dictates prognosis, we should have the maximum information to optimize management. There is little doubt that the young should have the aggressive approach, but with non-invasive screening being reliable, those with mild to moderate symptoms should only be evaluated by angiography if their treadmill ECG is strongly positive for significant coronary artery disease. Clearly the elderly should be managed on symptoms *but* they have a right to angiography and should not be discounted on age alone.

Modifying the risk

In the subsets already discussed we can see that we can identify those at risk and modify the risk where appropriate with surgery. The practical summary is illustrated in Figure 4.8.

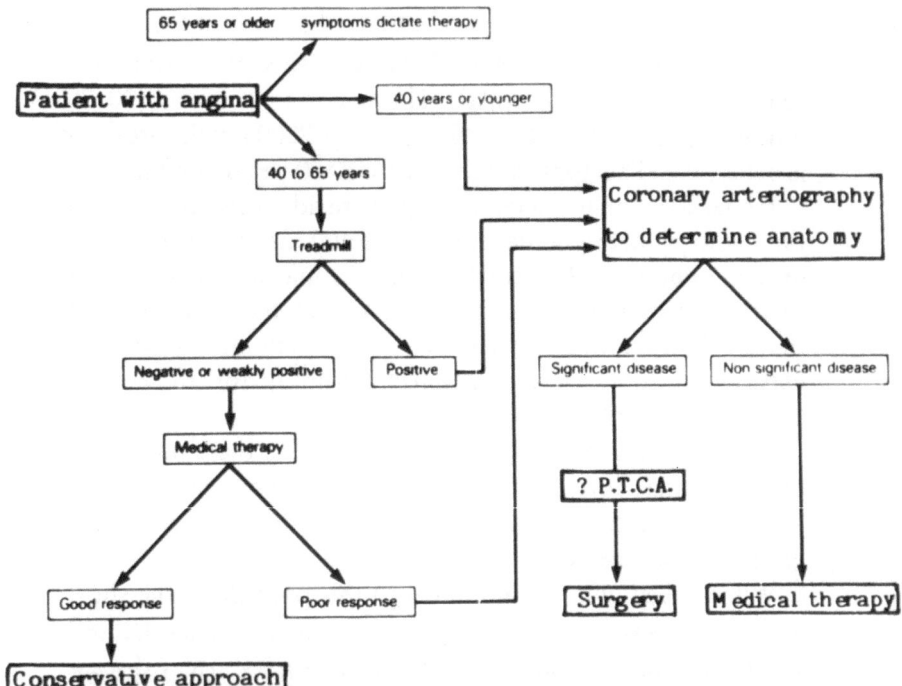

Figure 4.8 Investigations of the patient with stable angina

MANAGEMENT

Prevention in general

Prevention must be the prime objective of all involved in any aspect of medicine. The major risk factors can be either avoidable (e.g. smoking) or unavoidable (e.g. ageing). It is important to remember that risk factors are additive and that individuals with one or more risk factors should be pursued

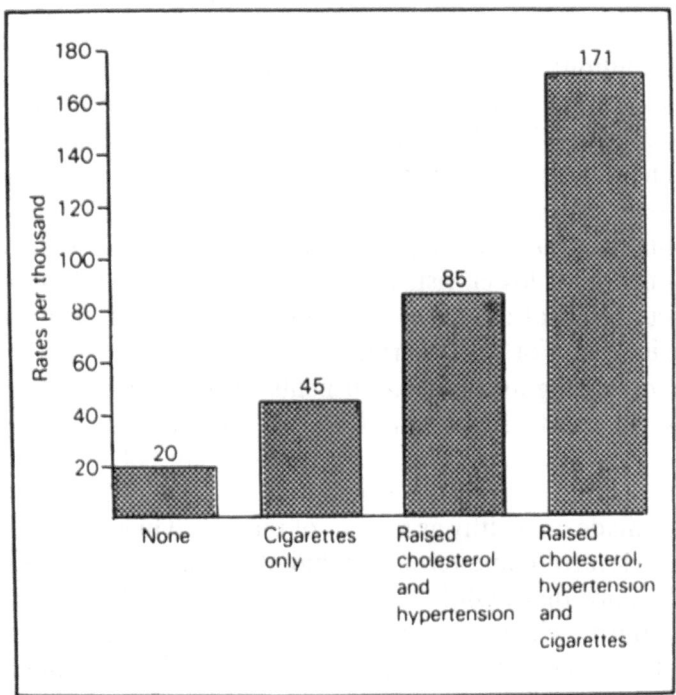

Figure 4.9   The additive effect of risk factors on the incidence of the first major coronary event

vigorously (Fig. 4.9). With the prospect of an additional 800 in 10 000 males reaching age 65 if primary prevention is successful, we can see a benefit both in the quality and quantity of life of the individual and cost to the community.

Results of the primary prevention trials have unfortunately been disappointing, apart from a reduction in coronary mortality from stopping smoking. Certainly eliminating smoking, eating a prudent diet, increasing dynamic exercise and avoiding obesity sound sensible but there is little evidence to support mass intervention, such as a change (compulsory?) in world-wide lifestyle[15].

Selective screening, focusing on high-risk individuals and their relatives, concentrates efforts and resources on far fewer people with the chance of greater impact on prevention. Here, in addition to smoking, there is a clear benefit from cholesterol lowering for those in the top quartile of serum cholesterol distribution[16]. However, only one study supports this philosophy – The Lipid Research Clinic's 'Coronary primary prevention trial (LRC)' of cholestyramine[17]. Studying the top 5% of cholesterol elevation, those treated had a 19% reduction in coronary deaths and non-fatal infarcts. However, confidence limits were poor, making it difficult to extend the intervention argument to lower risk groups. Indeed it is overlooked in discussion that in the treated group there was an increase in the incidence of oral gastrointestinal cancer.

Controlling hypertension benefits stroke incidence, but the data for mild to moderate hypertension and coronary heart disease is negative. The recent MRC trial[18] of mild hypertension demonstrated no benefit and 20–25% of healthy men were made unhealthy as a result of therapy. Thus, whilst those with elevated cholesterols and blood pressure are at risk, the risk is not that high because in men aged 40–55 years about two-thirds will be fit over the next 25 years without intervention[19]. This means that major lifestyle changes, lipid lowering agents and antihypertensives will in the majority have been unnecessary. However, the public are at the mercy of the marketing men and no scientific argument will overcome the commercial interest in developing and profiting from low cholesterol products.

Prevention: practical

We must not punish our patients or instill them with guilt. We must concentrate on reducing smoking, which is responsible for 25% of coronary deaths in those under 65 years and 80% of men below 45 years. Cigarettes increase the myocardial workload by catecholamine stimulation, at the same time as reducing oxygen supply by carbon monoxide inhalation. This combined with increased platelet adhesiveness is a recipe for disaster.

All smokers are at risk but especially those with additional risk factors such as hypertension or diabetes. The risks of a future infarct can be reduced by half within five years of stopping smoking[20] (Fig. 4.10).

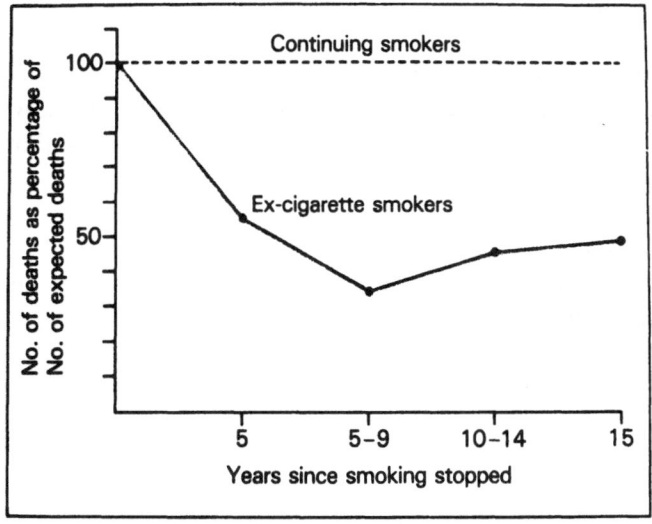

Figure 4.10 Mortality from coronary heart disease is halved five years after stopping smoking

General practical advice should emphasize the importance of annual blood pressure screening, regular exercise if enjoyed and avoidance of obesity because people close to optimal

> **General practical advice**
> - Stop smoking
> - Annual blood pressure screening
> - Regular exercise *if* enjoyed
> - Avoid obesity

weight feel better than when overweight. However, the slothful, who hate exercise should be told to stop smoking and left otherwise alone.

General advice

There is no substitute for a careful, clear explanation of the nature of the problem, the reasons it occurred and how the patient can help himself by modifying his risk status. Patients are often devastated by the diagnosis of a heart condition and time spent with them and their spouses is invaluable in putting the problems in perspective and guiding them forward positively. Booklets are available to reinforce the advice and to answer questions often forgotten at the interview.

Obesity

Obesity increases the workload of the heart and weight reduction can be an asset in pain control. We routinely advise on diet, using our dietitians frequently. It is important to remember that after stopping smoking many patients gain weight. At this time the patient should be reassured and it should be made clear that the greatest achievement is to stop smoking, advice on weight should follow later.

Regular exercise

This may improve the patient's well-being. Whilst there is no statistical evidence that regular exercise reduces morbidity or mortality, studies show a consistently favourable trend. It is important to emphasize the need to *enjoy* exercise. There is no point in jogging if you hate it, better to walk in the countryside. Isometric exercise (press-ups, weight training) should be avoided because of excessive heart rate and blood pressure rises. The main advantages of a treadmill ECG in assessing risk and the need for investigations have been stated previously; but a further use is in giving the patient confidence in what he can do, as well as guiding us or advising on his physical abilities. For example, a patient with mild angina and a good treadmill can safely go skiing.

Most people can maintain their *employment,* but heavy goods vehicle licences must be surrendered. Otherwise driving is safe. Stress is a problem in the presence of other risk factors, but not as an isolated entity. It is worth advising the patient to consider the emotionally demanding aspects of his lifestyle in the working and home environment. Regular holidays, non-stressful lunchtime and home activities (gardening, walking, reading) help complete a lifestyle change that the patient may find easier to follow than expected.

Type A individuals – ambitious, competitive, aggressive, impatient

These may be more at risk than their relaxed Type B counter-parts. Here it is of interest that beta-blockade can induce personality change from A to B, which may be useful in the appropriate patients with anginal pain[22].

Sexual activity

A question seldom asked concerns sexual activity. Stress on the heart during sex is no greater than during normal daily activity, providing the couples are married or have been cohabiting for some time. The casual relationship with its greater stress factor does lead to a more vigorous cardiovascular response. A useful practical guide is the rule of two flights of stairs. If the patient can briskly climb up and down two flights of stairs without symptoms, sex will most times be angina free. Extramarital sex is associated with a greater chance of cardiac event, but this may be preventable by specific drug therapy with nitrates and beta-blockade[23].

DRUG THERAPY

Nitrates

Nitrates are potent venodilators and to a lesser extent arterial dilators (Table 4.5). They benefit the symptoms of angina by lowering the workload of the heart secondary to vasodilatation. Coronary vasodilatation occurs to a variable extent but peripheral effects are responsible for the majority of the benefit. Nitrates can be used safely and effectively in addition to beta-blockade and calcium antagonists.

Sublingual glyceryl trinitrate (GTN) avoids hepatic metabolism and is effective in two to three minutes and may be repeated. It may be used for the relief of angina or prophylactically. GTN loses its potency after 2–3 months and should be stored if possible in a darkened glass bottle without cotton wool in a fridge. GTN spray delivers 400 micrograms with each jet spray, lasts up to three years but is more expensive. However, it may be advantageous when the patient's pain in infrequent. The principal side effect is headaches, about which all patients should be warned. GTN lasts up to 30 minutes sublingually and for a more prolonged effect, sublingual isosorbide dinitrate may be preferred (e.g. 5 mg before sexual intercourse).

Oral nitrates have, until recently, relied on hepatic metabolism converting the dinitrate to its active metabolite, the mononitrate. This has led to substantial variability in effect

Table 4.5 Nitrate preparations

Preparation	Use	Problems
Sublingual GTN	Alleviate attacks quickly; prophylaxis 30 minutes	Headaches. Replenish every 2–3 months. Careful storage
GTN spray (400 µg)	Alleviate attacks quickly; prophylaxis 30 minutes	Expensive. Headaches. Inflammable
Topical nitrates	Nocturnal symptoms? Debatable any use	Expensive, short duration of action, patch cosmetically better than paste
Isosorbide dinitrate:		
1. Sublingual	Prophylaxis one hour	As GTN
2. Oral	Prevention of pain. 10–40 mg bid	Hepatic metabolism + Tolerance +
Isosorbide mononitrate	Prevention of pain. 10–40 mg bid	Early results encouraging. 100% bio-availability
Buccal nitrates	Alleviate pain and prophylaxis	Expensive, not well tolerated

from patient to patient. In addition, tolerance (decreased effect with time) has been reported within days[24]. The development of isosorbide mononitrate offers 100% bioavailability and clinical trials are most encouraging concerning its effectiveness and lack of tolerance[25]. Our current recommendation is isosorbide mononitrate 10 mg bid, increasing to 20 mg bid and 40 mg bid occasionally.

Buccal glyceryl trinitrate offers the advantage of immediate release of nitrate, though slower than GTN, with a more gradual release over four hours or so. It appears to be effective, variably tolerated, but expensive. It may be of value when oral medication is not possible, as in the pre-operative or post-operative state.

Topical nitrates were developed to avoid hepatic metabolism but have proved a disappointing and expensive failure. I consider them only of value for nocturnal pain or breathlessness because of the very short duration of action[26].

Occasionally, as well as headaches, nitrates can cause postural hypotension, though this is more common in the elderly. Taken overall they are the safest of all anti-anginal preparations and can be used in heart failure, where a haemodynamic benefit may also be achieved.

Beta-blockade

Beta-adrenergic blockade reduces sympathetically mediated increases in heart rate, systolic blood pressure and myocardial contractility and thereby reduces myocardial demand. These actions, produced by competition at the beta-adrenergic receptors, lead to a reduction in angina attacks and the need for GTN as well as an increase in exercise tolerance with less ischaemia on the electrocardiogram. Furthermore, the number of ischaemic episodes over 24 hours, whether silent or not, are reduced[27, 28]. Beta-blockade is effective in over 90% of patients.

In Table 4.6 the individual agents and properties are summarized. Some are cardioselective in that they preferentially block β_1-receptors in the heart, rather than β_2 in the lungs or blood vessels. These are less likely to produce problems by blocking sympathetically mediated bronchodilation and peripheral vasodilation, as well as being less likely to impair glucose release in response to hypoglycaemia. They will, however, mask the tachycardia the diabetic may be using as a warning sign. Selectivity is *relative* and decreases with increasing dosage of each agent. Where doubt exists I would select a calcium antagonist.

Some agents (e.g. pindolol or acebutolol) have partial agonist activity and are theoretically less likely to produce extremes of bradycardia, bronchoconstriction or vasoconstriction. In patients with severe angina, this may be a disadvantage

Table 4.6 A practical approach to selecting a beta-blocker for angina[a]

	Potency	Cardio-selective	Optimum dose dynamic half-life (hours)	Blood-brain barrier penetration	Doseage adjustments
Acebutolol	0.3	±[b]	24	NS	Renal
Atenolol	1	+	24	NS	Renal
Metoprolol	1	+	10–12	Yes	Liver
Nadolol	1.5	0	39	NS	Renal
Oxprenolol	0.5–1	0	13	Yes	Liver
Pindolol	6	0	8	Yes	None
Propranolol	1	0	8	Yes++	Liver
Sotalol	0.3	0	24	NS	Renal
Timolol	6	0	15	Yes	Liver
Slow oxprenolol			<24		
Metoprolol SA			24		
Propranolol LA			24		

[a] *How to use this table:* Assume propranolol as the reference drug with a potency of one. Propranolol 80 mg can be given twice daily (half-life 11 hours). It is equal to atenolol 100 mg (potency 1:1) and atenolol can be given once daily (half-life 24 hours). Sotalol is one-third the potency of propranolol so that it needs to be given 240 mg once daily to be equivalent to propranolol 80 mg bid, i.e. we compare dosage to 80 mg propranolol equivalent, *not* to total daily dose.

[b] Cardioselectivity of acebutolol is debated.

NS = not significant.

because of lack of effect on the resting heart rate; whereas in those with peripheral side effects, the less depressant effect on cardiac output may substantially reduce the problems of coldness and heaviness of the limbs.

In general, beta-blockers are well tolerated and remain first line drugs in the treatment of angina pectoris. Beta-blockade is competitive and the major reason for a poor response remains a failure to give enough medication. Because of the varying potencies of individual beta-blockers, it is important to be thoroughly familiar with the use of one or two agents (Table 4.6).

Whilst caution is advised in commencing beta-blockade (low doses initially, so that side effects can be easily reversed), it is important to titrate dose to effect. In general, the average dose is equivalent to propranolol 80 mg bid or tds, e.g. atenolol 100 mg daily (see Table 4.6)[29].

Adverse effects are largely predictable and often caused by inappropriate patient selection. Why give someone with bronchospasm a cardioselective beta-blocker when there is a chance of problems, when a nitrate or calcium antagonist will avoid that chance? Bronchospasm and heart failure are well recognized adverse effects, but cold hands and feet, heavy legs, lethargy and a general washed-out feeling are more frequently experienced. These symptoms reflect a fall in cardiac output, which is common to all beta-blockers, so that they may improve with dosage reduction or transfer to an agent with ISA (e.g. acebutolol). Central nervous system side effects – such as muzzy head, loss of memory, poor concentration, vivid dreams and depression – also occur and seem to be related to blood-brain passage, which is a greater problem with the lipid soluble (lipophilic) agents. Using a hydrophilic agent (water soluble) these effects may be substantially reduced or even abolished. Noting the mode of excretion of individual beta-blockers the obvious dose adjustments can be anticipated in patients with significant renal or hepatic disease. Similarly, drug interactions may be anticipated if two drugs excreted via hepatic metabolism are used, e.g. propranolol and cimetidine.

Calcium antagonists

Calcium ions are essential for myocardial contraction and conduction. Calcium antagonists act by impairing the influx of these ions into smooth muscle, myocardial and conducting tissue cells. The three agents available are nifedipine, diltiazem and verapamil. All act as peripheral vasodilators but individual important differences exist (Table 4.7). In therapeutic doses, though they only have a mild effect on cardiac contractility, they must still be used with caution in patients with impaired left ventricular function – especially in the presence of beta-blockade.

Table 4.7   The calcium antagonists

	Nifedipine	*Verapamil*	*Diltiazem*
Heart rate	↑	↓↑	↓↑
AV conduction	0	↓↓	↓
Peripheral vasodilation	+ + +	+ +	+ +
Coronary vasodilation	+ + +	+ +	+ + +
Contractility	↓0	↓↓	↓

Verapamil

This has a marked action on the atrioventricular node and is consequently a powerful antiarrhythmic drug, particularly for supraventricular tachycardias. In several studies it has been shown to be just as effective as beta-blockade in stable angina pectoris[30]. It is not recommended for co-prescribing with beta-blockade because the additive effect on AV conduction can induce asystole or heart block. It is of great value in patients with obstructive airways disease or peripheral arterial disease, where beta-blockade may be contraindicated. It is effective in doses of 40 mg tds increasing to 120 mg tds. Principal side effects are flushing and headaches secondary to vasodilatation and constipation (especially in the elderly).

Nifedipine

This is a potent arterial vasodilator with no effect on AV conduction. It is therefore a safe drug to use in combination with beta-blockade.

Its use as a single agent in angina is surprisingly poorly documented. The possibility of a reflex tachycardia or coronary steal effect renders the need for caution in its use. Several reports detail the need for individual dose titration and the difficulty in giving guidelines for drug useage[31], its failure in the smoking population[32], and the overall superiority of beta blockade in comparison[33]. However, the additive effect to beta-blockade is clear and this is where I believe its use lies in stable angina. Typical doses are 5 mg tds increasing to 40 mg bid.

Diltiazem

This is a relatively new agent, very similar in profile to Verapamil. Though it possesses effects on AV conduction, its use in combination with beta-blockade has been reported to be safe[34]. However, I would still urge caution at this early stage, particularly as nifedipine avoids any risk. Its clinical effectiveness in stable angina has been established but it remains to be seen whether its reportedly reduced side effect profile (less flushing, less constipation) is maintained with widespread use. Typical dose is 60 mg tds and it can be used as monotherapy as an alternative to beta blockade[35].

Combination therapy

Though we have only three groups of drugs, no data is available on which is better than which in combination. There is no doubt that calcium antagonists together with nitrates are safe and triple therapy using nifedipine is safe. However, angina needing this amount of drug control should be investigated further to see if a surgical option is possible (Fig. 4.11).

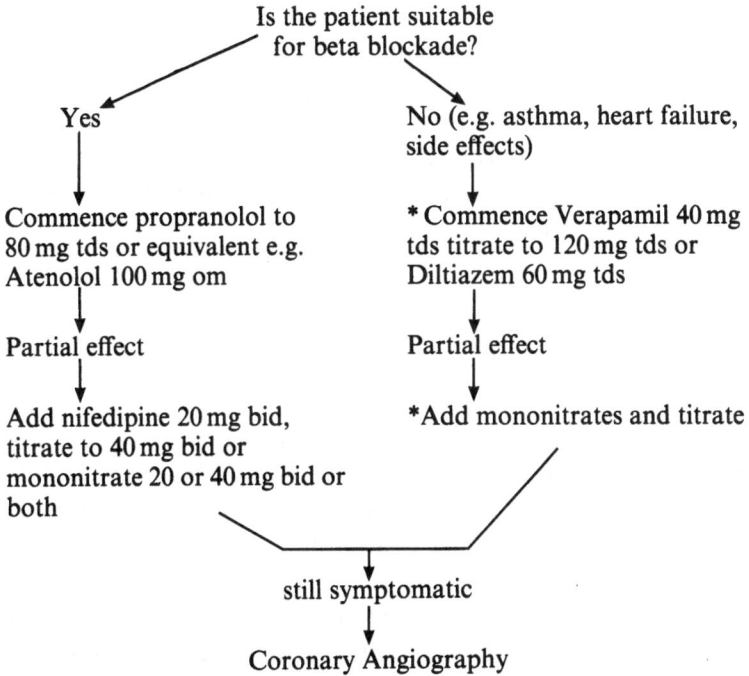

Figure 4.11   Medical treatment of stable angina

ANGIOPLASTY

Percutaneous transluminal coronary angioplasty (PCTA) has given the physician for the first time, the possibility to increase the supply of blood to the heart rather than reduce the demand[36]. Unfortunately, in our excitement, we have failed to control our observations and failed to provide satisfactory comparisons with conventional medical therapy or bypass surgery. In 1985 60000 angioplasties were performed in the USA with no-one knowing if they were providing optimal therapy.

The procedure is similar to coronary angiography. The stenosis is identified, a guide wire passed over it and a balloon advanced along the guide wire until it crosses the lesion. The balloon is than inflated and hopefully the stenosis substantially reduced (Figs. 4.12, 4.13). Currently reported initial success rates are 90%, with a recurrence rate at six months of 20–30%. The procedure can then be repeated with a further 80% success rate. As no comparative data exists regarding bypass surgery, I have had to use historical controls from surgical publications.

In single vessel disease there is no difference from surgery initially but surgery is better at 12 months (Table 4.8) symtomatically. The problem here is that we know medical therapy alone is successful in single vessel disease[5, 6] and we must assume PTCA is frequently being performed, based on the 'looks' of the lesion and not the symptoms of the patient.

In multivessel disease (Table 4.9), the results are not as impressive when scrutinized carefully, despite the enthusiasm of the PTCA protagonists[37].

Clearly we are in desperate need of a randomized controlled trial of PTCA and bypass surgery in patients with stable angina. Obviously, if PTCA is shown to be as good as surgery in various subsets, it will offer a far less painful therapeutic

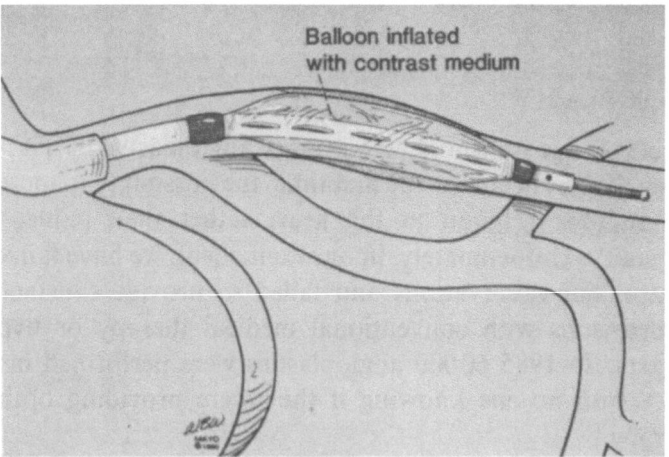

Balloon inflated
with contrast medium

Figure 4.12   PTCA balloon advanced

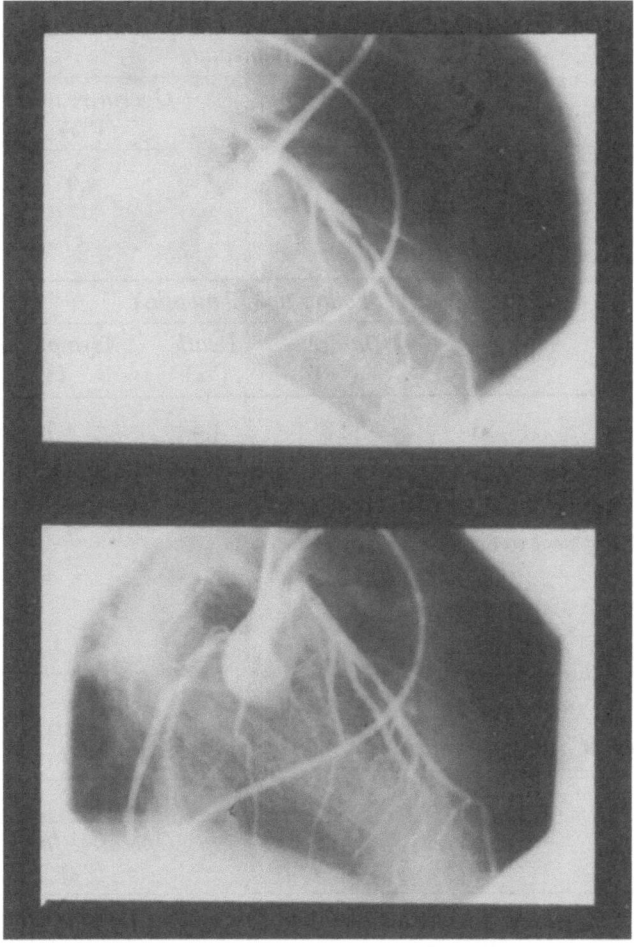

Figure 4.13 Successful angioplasty: (top) critical stenosis; (bottom) after dilatation

option for the patient. In the meanwhile, patients with symptoms and single or multivessel disease involving short (< 2 cm) lesions should be considered for PTCA – but only if they are provided with an honest appraisal of plusses and minuses and the advantages and disadvantages of the surgical option.

Table 4.8   Surgery versus PTCA in single vessel disease

	Immediate		
	Success (%)	*Death* (%)	*Operative infarct* (%)
PTCA	90 (CABG 6.5)	1	4.9
Surgery	N/A	1	3

	Follow up (*12 months*)			
	Re-op (%)	*Infarct* (%)	*Death* (%)	*Asymptomatic* (%)
PTCA	15 (12 CABG)	2.8	1.4	70
Surgery	3	1.5	< 3	90

NB. Equivalent to medical therapy alone.

Table 4.9   Surgery versus PTCA in multivessel disease[37]

	Immediate		
	Success (%)	*Death* (%)	*Operative Infarct* (%)
PTCA	92 (CABG 1)	1.2	3–5
Surgery	N/A	< 2.0	< 5

	Follow up (*12 months*)			
	Re-op (%)	*Infarct* (%)	*Death* (%)	*Asymptomatic* (%)
PTCA	27 (15 CABG)	7.3	5.6	64
Surgery	3	1.5	3	80

SURGERY

1. Stable angina

The role of surgery in stable angina for relief of symptoms and to lengthen life is well established[5, 6]. It is effective in all age groups and those otherwise fit but over 65 years benefit as well as the younger patients[38]. In experienced hands, the operative mortality is less than 2% and approximately three months after the procedure, a normal lifestyle should be possible. Musculoskeletal pain and leg pain from the vein site may

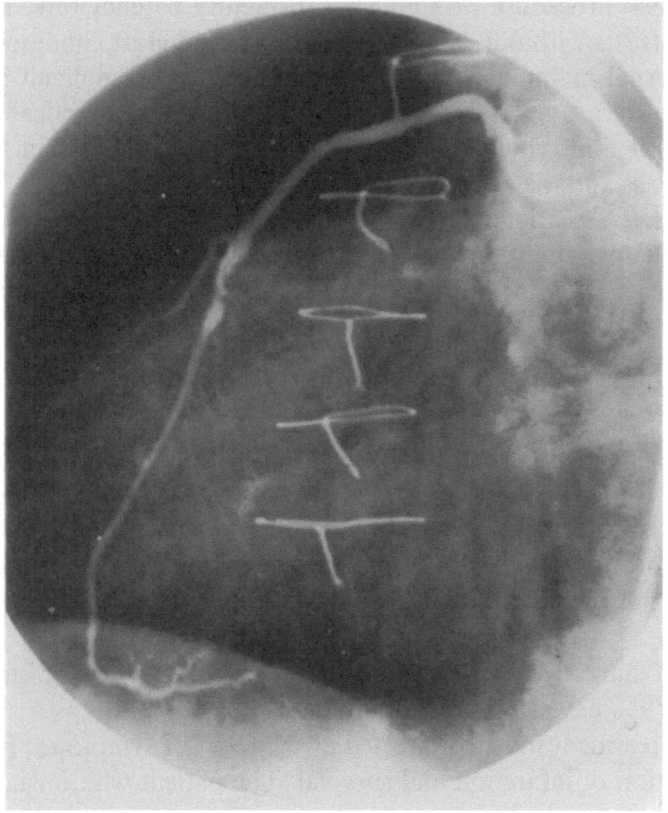

Figure 4.14 Successful bypass surgery

persist for several weeks and require regular analgesia or anti-inflammatory agents.

The major concern is the longterm effectiveness of the bypass operation (Fig. 4.14). Attention to risk factors is essential and in the first 12 months antiplatelet therapy is also used with either dipyridamole plus aspirin or aspirin alone[39]. In this way, 12 month patency is of the order of 85–90%. However, atheroma is a relentless disease and surgery bypasses but does not cure the problem.

Ten-year follow-up has demonstrated very encouraging results when the internal mammary artery is employed for the bypass procedure with a 95% satisfactory patency rate. This contrasts with only a 50% satisfactory vein graft condition[40]. Internal mammary grafting is technically more difficult and the artery less suitable in the elderly, so, given the practicalities of life, the young, where possible, should undergo artery bypass and the elderly vein bypass.

It is essential to monitor risk factors after surgery with particular attention being paid to smoking, weight control and hypertension supervision (the surgeon often overlooks these!).

2. Unstable angina

The mechanism for the development of unstable angina may be: an external aggravation of a stable condition (e.g. emotional shock); progression of atheroma or plaque rupture; or coronary vasoconstriction (spasm). Ten percent or less have normal or minimally diseased arteries in which spasm must play a part – approximately 20% have single vessel disease, 27% have two vessel disease, 44% have three vessel disease and 9% have left main stem disease[41].

Treatment must be directed at the relief of symptoms, prevention of infarction and survival. The patient with unstable angina should be commenced on nitrates and immediately admitted to the local Coronary Care Unit. In the unit, conventional analgesia is introduced with diamorphine and intravenous nitrate therapy commenced and titrated to effect. In those in whom it is not contraindicated, beta-blockade without ISA should be commenced; and in the others oral diltiazem or verapamil but not nifedipine should be given. Nifedipine can be added to beta-blockade for further effect and nitrates added orally as the intravenous line is tailed off. Failure to stabilize therapy with drugs is unusual but the intra-aortic balloon pump can then be utilized in specialized centres. Aspirin should be commenced 300 mg daily[42] because of a clear cut protective effect against acute myocardial infarction.

If symptoms continue, either emergency surgery or PTCA should be considered, but again there is no trial between the two[43]. Providing medical stabilization occurs, the prognosis in the short term is favourable, but in view of a subsequent infarct rate of up to 15% at 4 months and 12 month mortality of 10%, routine angiography is advised when the patient has been fully stabilized for a few days. If then considered anatomically at risk, successful results are achieved from elective

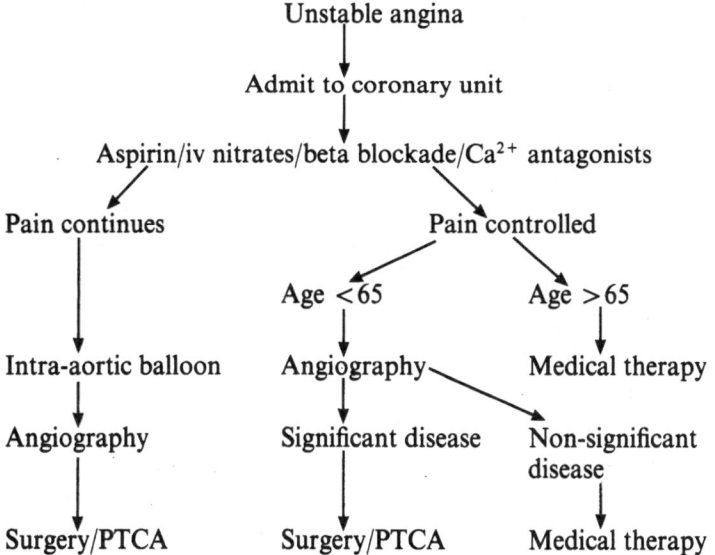

Figure 4.15   Unstable angina management plan

bypass surgery with a 61% ten year asymptomatic rate, 20% minimally symtomatic, 14% suffering angina on ordinary effort and 5% severe angina. The operative mortality is 1.8% with a 10 year survival rate of 83%[44]. A treatment strategy is summarized in Figure 4.15.

3. Variant angina (spasm)

Spasm with ST elevation can occur in the presence or absence of fixed atheromatous coronary artery disease. Treatment involves nitrates and calcium antagonists[35, 45]. The natural history has not been extensively studied but a high complication rate with infarction and sudden death is recognized. Vasospastic angina is not clearly defined or understood, making the management a subject for specialist centres rather than outpatient practice. It does not form greater than 5% of clinical practice.

CHEST PAIN WITH NORMAL CORONARY ARTERIES

When the investigation reveals no obstructive lesion, the first thing to do is to emphatically reassure the patient. The second thing to do is retake the history. It may have been atypical originally but now it is time to check for musculoskeletal problems or oesophageal symptoms. A significant number may have the hyperventilation syndrome and respiratory function tests and physiotherapy may be curative.

The scientific trap the cardiologist falls into is to pursue other options, such as cardiac biopsy or metabolic studies, which reinforce in the patient's mind that he is abnormal. This can lead to mistrust in the doctor, particularly when the patient has been told there is no obvious problem in the coronary arteries. Just by being told they are normal an improvement may occur but if the symptoms continue and none of the above are proven to cause the pain, I believe a formal psychiatric assessment should precede any other therapeutic option. To blame spasm as the cause is to avoid the difficulties of unravelling the problems of many individuals. For the small number in whom no other cause can be found, a trial of calcium antagonists or nitrates is indicated. I believe it is imperative that these people are not put repeatedly through more complex cardiological investigations that will only achieve one end result – the doctor gains scientific satisfaction, but the patient develops chronic hypochondriasis.

Useful practical points

- Angina is a clinical diagnosis made on symptoms
- Unstable angina is new or worsening angina with the development of rest pain – it is a dangerous condition and routine coronary angiography is advised in these patients
- Exercise testing may be helpful in diagnosing patients with chest pain but coronary arteriography is the definitive test and should be considered in all anginal patients below 40 years of age to decide whether operation is desirable
- There is little evidence to support a radical change in life-style in order to prevent coronary artery disease
- GP advice should emphasize stopping smoking, avoidance of obesity and the need for regular exercise; an annual BP check may also be helpful
- Nitrates, beta-blockers and calcium antagonists remain the mainstay of symptomatic control of angina
- If a coronary arteriogram is normal in a patient with chest pain, always reassure the patient, then retake the history and look for non-cardiac causes

REFERENCES

1. Heberden, W. (1772). Some account of a disorder of the breast. Read at the Royal College of Physicians July 1768., *Med. Trans. Coll. Physicians*, **2**, 59–67
2. Sampson, J.J. and Cheitlin, M.D. (1971). Pathophysiology and differential diagnosis of cardiac pain. *Prog. Cardiovasc. Dis.*, **13**, 507
3. Lichtlen, P.R. (1985). Pathophysiology of coronary and myocardial function in angina pectoris: important aspects for drug treatment. *Eur. Heart J.*, **5** (Suppl. F) 11–25
4. Prinzmetal, M. Kennamer, R., Merliss, R., Wade, T. and Bor, N. (1959). Angina Pectoris I. A variant form of angina pectoris. *Am. J. Med.* **27**, 375–88
5. European Coronary Surgery Study Group (1982). Long-term results of prospective randomised study of coronary artery bypass surgery in stable angina pectoris. *Lancet*, **ii**, 1173–80
6. CASS principal Investigators and Associates (1983). Coronary artery surgery study (CASS): a randomized trial of coronary artery bypass surgery: survival data. *Circ.*, **68**, 939–50
7. CASS (1983). A randomized trial of coronary artery bypass surgery: quality of life in patients randomly assigned to treatment groups. *Circ.*, **68**, 951–60
8. Passamani, E., Davis, K.B., Gillespie, M.J. and Killip, T. (1985). A randomised trial of coronary artery bypass surgery. *N. Eng. J. Med.*, **312**, 1665–71
9. Froelicher, F.V., Thomas, M.M., Pillow, C. and Lancaster, M.C. (1974). Epidemiological study of asymptomatic men screened by maximum treadmill testing for latent coronary artery disease. *Am. J. Cardiol.*, **34**, 770
10. Ellestad, M.H., Cooke, M.M. Jr. and Greenberg, P.S. (1979). Stress testing: clinical application and predictive capacity. *Prog. Cardiovasc. Dis.*, **21**, 431–60
11. Rochmis, P., Blackburn, H. (1971). Exercise tests: A survey of procedures, safety and litigation experience in approximately 170,000 tests. *J. Am. Med. Assoc.*, **217**, 1061
12. Ritchie, J.L., Trobaugh, G.B., Hamilton, G.W., Gould, K.L., Narahara, K.A., Murray, J.A., and Williams, D.L. (1977). Myocardial imaging with Thallium-201 at rest and during exercise. Comparison with coronary arteriography and resting and stress electrocardiography. *Circ.*, **56**, 66–71
13. Borer, J.S., Kent, K.M., Bacharach, S.L. (1979). Sensitivity, specificity and predictive accuracy of radionuclide cineangiography during exercise in patients with coronary artery disease. *Circ.*, **60**, 752–80
14. Davis, K., Kennedy, J.W. and Kemp, H.G. Jr. (1979). Complications of coronary arteriography from the collaborative study of coronary artery surgery (CASS). *Circ.*, **59**, 1105–12
15. Oliver, M.F. (1985). Strategies for preventing and screening for coronary heart disease. *Br. Heart J.*, **54**, 1–2

16. Report (1985). Consensus Conference: Lowering blood cholesterol to prevent heart disease. *J. Am. Med. Assoc.*, **253**, 2080
17. Lipid Research Clinics (1984) Coronary primary prevention trial i: Reduction in incidence of coronary heart disease. ii: The relationship of reduction in incidence of coronary heart disease to cholesterol lowering. *J. Am. Med. Assoc.*, **251**, 351
18. MRC (1985). Trial of treatment of mild hypertension: principal results. *Br. Med. J.*, **291**, 97
19. The Pooling Project Research Group (1978). Relationship of blood pressure, serum cholesterol, smoking habits, relative weight and ECG abnormalities to incidence of major coronary events. *J. Chron. Dis.*, **31**, 201
20. Doll, R. and Peto, R. (1976). Mortality in relation to smoking: 20 years observations on male doctors. *Br. Med. J.*, **2**, 1525–36.
21. Bass, C. (1983). Stress, personality and coronary heart disease. *Cardiol. Practice.*, **1**, 6–11
22. Schmeider R., Friedrich G., Neus, H., Rudel, H. and Von Eiff, A.W. (1983). The influence of beta-blockers on cardiovascular reactivity and type A behaviour pattern in hypertensives. *Psychosom. Med.*, **45**, 417–23
23. Jackson G. (1986). Cardiovascular response to sexual arousal and orgasm. *Br. J. Sex. Med.*, **13**, 8–9.
24. Thadani, U., Mangori, D., Parker, J.O., Fung, H.L. (1980). Tolerance to the effects of oral isosorbide dinitrate: Rate of development and cross tolerance to glyceryl trinitrate. *Circ.*, **61**, 526–35
25. Akhras, F., Jefferies, S. and Jackson, G. (1985). isosorbide-5-Mononitrate-effective monotherapy in chronic stable angina. *Zeitschrift kardiol.*, **74**, Supp 4, 16–20.
26. Editorial (1985). Transdermal nitrates: effective or not. *Lancet*, **ii**, 594–5
27. Jackson, G., Harry, J.D., Robinson, C., Kitson, D. and Jewitt, D.E. (1978). Comparison of atenolol with propranolol in the treatment of angina pectoris with special reference to once daily administration of atenolol. *Br. Heart J.*, **60**, 998–1004.
28. Jackson, G., Schwartz, J., Kates R.E., Winchester, M. and Harrison, D.C. (1980). Atenolol: Once daily cardioselective beta blockade for angina pectoris. *Circ.*, **61**, 555–60
29. Jackson, G., Atkinson, L. and Oram, S. (1975). Reassessment of failed beta blocker treatment in angina pectoris by peak exercise heart rate measurements. *Br. Med. J.*, **3**, 616–9.
30. Livesley, B., Catley, P.F., Campbell, R.C. and Oram, S. (1973). Double blind evaluation of verapamil, propranolol and isosorbide dinitrate against placebo in the treatment of angina pectoris. *Br. Med. J.*, **ii**, 375–8
31. Deanfield, J., Wright, C., Fox, K. (1983). Treatment of angina pectoris with nifedipine: importance of dose titration. *Br. Med. J.*, **286**, 1467–70
32. Deanfield, J., Wright, C., Krikler, S., Ribiero, P., Fox, K. (1984).

Cigarette smoking and the treatment of angina with propranolol, atenolol and nifedipine. *N. Eng. J. Med.,* **310,** 951–4.

33. Lynch, P., Dargie, H., Krikler, S., Krikler D. (1980) Objective assessment of antianginal treatment: a double blind comparison of propranolol, nifedipine and their combination. *Br. Med. J.,* **281,** 184–7.

34. Kenny, J., Daly, K., Bergman, G., Kerkez, S., Jewitt, D.E. (1985). Beneficial effects of diltiazem combined with beta blockade in angina pectoris. *Eur. Heart J.,* **6,** 418–23

35. Chaffman, M., Brogden, R.N. (1985). Diltiazem: A review of its pharmacological properties and therapeutic efficacy. *Drugs,* **29,** 387–454

36. Editorial (1985). The expanding scope of coronary angioplasty. *Lancet,* **i,** 1307–8

37. Hartzler, G.O. (1985). Complex coronary angioplasty: an alternative therapy. *Int. J. Cardiol,* **9,** 133–7

38. CASS (1985). Comparison of coronary artery bypass surgery and medical therapy in patients 65 years of age or older. *N. Eng. J. Med.,* **9,** 133–7

39. Chesebro, J.H. et al. (1984). Effect of dipyridamole and aspirin on late vein graft patency after coronary bypass operation. *N. Eng. J. Med.,* **310,** 209–14

40. Editorial (1986). The internal mammary artery: the ideal coronary bypass graft. *N. Eng. J. Med.,* **314,** 50–51

41. Rahimtoola, S.H., Nunley, D., Grunkemeier, G., Tepley, J., Lambert, L., Starr, A. (1983). Ten year survival after coronary bypass surgery for unstable angina. *N. Engl. J. Med.,* **308,** 676–81

42. Lewis, H.D., et al. (1983). Protective effects of aspirin against acute myocardial infarction and death in men with unstable angina. *N. Engl. J. Med.,* **309,** 396–403

43. De Feyter, P.J., Serruys, P.W., Van den Brand, M., Balakumaran, K., Mochtar, B., Soward, A.L., Arnold, A.E.R., Hugenholtz, P.G. (1985). Emergency coronary angioplasty in refractory unstable angina. *N. Engl. J. Med.,* **313,** 342–6

44. Rahimtoola, S.H. (1984). Coronary bypass surgery for unstable angina. *Circ.,* **69,** 842–8

45. Johnson, S.M., Mauritson, D.R., Willerson, J.T., Hillis, L.D. (1981). A controlled trial of verapamil for prinzmetal's angina. *N. Engl. J. Med.,* **304,** 862–6

INDEX

Note: The following abbreviations have been used in subdivisions in this index: CCU – coronary care unit; CHD – coronary heart disease.

acebutolol 110, 111, 112
Action on Smoking and Health,
    address 57
airway maintenance, in cardiac
    arrest 12
alcohol intake reduction
    as preventive measure 30
    in management of hypertension 37
ambulance crew training 11
ambulances 11
amiloride 19
aminophylline 14
anaemia 93
    in stable angina 94
analgesics 9
    see also drug therapy
angina
    aetiology 93–4
    causes 91
    character of pain 88–90
    clinical effects 86–7
    coronary angiography 17, 121
    diagnosis 85
    differential diagnosis 7–8
    late complication of myocardial
        infarction 18–19
    management 53

nature of pain 87–90
need for exercise training 81
pain at night 91
pain relief 91–2
prevention 103–6
radiation of pain 88
results of exercise testing 64, 70
site of pain 87–8
stable 86–92
    assessment 94–8
    auscultatory findings 94
    drug therapy 108–15
    identification of patients at
        risk 98–102
    investigations 95
    management 103–8
    modifying risk 102
    role of surgery 119–20
    those at risk 95–8
treatment 19
unstable 92
    drug therapy 120–1
    mechanisms 120
    surgical treatment 121–2
variant 92–3
    treatment 122
angiography *see* coronary angiography

angioplasty *see* percutaneous
        transluminal coronary
        angioplasty (PTCA)
anticoagulants   14–15, 21, 53
aortic dissection, pain of   8
aortic stenosis   93
arcus senilis, in hyperlipidaemia   94
arrhythmias   12
    as cause of death   1
    in heart attacks   6
    management   10
    monitoring in CCUs   13
    post-infarction treatment   52
    temporary pacing   20
    treatment   20
arterial embolism, complicating heart
        attack   12
aspirin   53, 121
atenolol   10, 19, 111
atrial fibrillation   20
atropine   10

bed rest   15
    effects   65–6
bendrofluazide   19
beta-blockers   10, 53, 110–12
    adverse effects   112
    arrhythmia treatment   20
    avoidance before exercise testing   80
    beneficial in post-hospital
        management   22
    of angina   19
    for unstable angina   121
    in combination therapy   114–15
blood pressure
    annual screening   44, 105, 106
    during heart attacks   6
    exercise-induced changes   17
    in aortic dissection   8
bradycardia, management of   10
brain damage, from cardiac arrest   11
breast feeding, benefits   46–7
breathing, artificial respiration   12
    see also airway maintenance
breathlessness, in heart attack   6
British Heart Foundation, address   57
Bruce protocol   68
buprenorphine   9

calcium antagonists   53. 113–14
    angina control   19
    combination therapy   114–15

cardiac arrest
    management   11–12
    symptoms   11
cardiac enlargement   63
cardiac rhythm, ECG monitoring   7
    see also arrhythmias
Chest, Heart and Stroke Association,
        address   57
chest pain
    differential diagnosis   85–6
    nature, in angina   87
    with normal coronary arteries   122–
        3
    see also pain
cholesterol levels   20–1
    benefits of reduction   104
    normal   44–5
    reduction, in secondary CHD
        prevention   52
    risk factor in CHD   2, 35–6, 63
    screening   44
cimetidine   112
circuit training   74, 80
circulation, maintenance, in cardiac
        arrest   12
compression, to maintain
        circulation   12
coronary angiography   17, 61, 64
    cost   101
    for under-40-year-olds   98
    in unstable angina   121
    mortality rate   101
    procedure   101
    referral after exercise training   74, 80
    suitability of patient   101–2
coronary artery bypass grafting   17–18,
        23, 61, 65
    compared with angioplasty   116, 118
    following unsuccessful drug
        therapy   19
    results   120
    use of exercise training   81
Coronary Artery Disease Research
        Association (CORDA),
        address   57
Coronary Artery Surgical Study
        (CASS)   96–8
coronary care units (CCUs)
    duration of stay   15
    handling other diseases   13
    monitoring arrhythmias   13
coronary heart disease   64
    causative factors   30

causing angina 91
comparison of UK with other
  countries 29
pattern 31
preventive measures 41
  strategy in general practice 42–6
progress 65
reduced incidence 28
reduced mortality in ex-smokers 105
risk factors 31, 35–41, 62–3
  additive effect 103
  role of family history 41
secondary prevention 49–54
  risk factors 50–2
  see also heart attacks
coronary insufficiency, acute 92
coronary thrombosis 1
counselling
  in CHD prevention 42–3
  in secondary CHD prevention 50
crescendo angina 92
cycle ergometers 68, 80

defibrillators
  in ambulance 11
  in CCUs 13
diabetes 12–13
diamorphine 9, 10, 14, 120
diet
  advice 78
  changes 30
    to reduce cholesterol levels 36, 45
  control, in secondary CHD
    prevention 50–1
  family 47
digoxin 20
diltiazem 113, 114, 121
Dindevan 21
dipyridamole 53
disopyramide 21
diuretics, in heart failure
    management 14, 19
driving 79
  limitations following heart
    attack 16–17, 53, 61, 107
drug therapy
  hypertension 37–8
  stable angina 108–15
  unstable angina 120–1

ECG
  during exercise testing 68, 70, 74
  in angina diagnosis 85

normal, in early heart attack 6–7
remote monitoring 15, 74
serial 75, 78
employment see heart attacks: return to
    work
European Coronary Surgery
    Study 95–6, 98
exercise
  advice 107
    on targets 78–9
  as preventive measure 30
  enjoyment 105–6, 107
  in rehabilitation 60, 62
  lack, risk factor in CHD 2, 31, 63
  post-heart attack 16
  to control hypertension 37
exercise testing 17, 18, 61, 98
  assessment 80
    for rehabilitation 63
  in Selly Oak scheme 79
  maximum oxygen uptake 70
  methods 68
  mortality and complications 100
  principles 67–8
  revealing residual disease 64
  significant endpoints 99–100
  symptom-limited maximum load 70
  see also treadmill testing
exercise training 71–3, 80–1
  programme 73–5
eyes, pupil abnormalities in cardiac
    arrest 11

facilitators, use in formulating
    preventive strategies 43
family health care 46–7
family history 2
fibre, dietary 36
fibrillation
  atrial 20
  ventricular 21, 100
fibrinolytic system 22–3
flecainide 20
follow-up 17–18
  in Selly Oak scheme 77–8
frusemide 10, 19, 20

general practitioners (GPs)
  communicating with hospital 78, 79
  encouraging non-smoking 32–3
  role in heart attacks 4
    long-term management 4, 16

general practitioners (GPs) – *cont.*
  role in preventive medicine   32–4
    strategy   42–6
glyceryl trinitrate   18–19, 91, 108,
    109

Health Education Council, address   57
health promotion literature   45–6
heart attacks
  death rate   2
  definition   1
  diagnosis   5–7
  differential diagnosis   7–9
  duration of hospitalization   62
  epidemiology   2
  follow-up   17–18
  future management trends   22–3
  immediate management   9–10
  incidence of home care   4
  management in hospital   12–16
  post-hospital phase   16–18
  prognosis   2–3
  return to normal life   53
  return to work   16–17, 53, 67, 78
  risk factors   2
  role of GP   4
  secondary prevention   20–2
  see also coronary heart disease
heart failure   12, 63
  induced by antiarrhythmic drugs   22
  late complication of myocardial
    infarction   19
  management in hospital   14
  reparable defects   61
  symptoms   6
Heberden, William   86–7
hospital admission   10
  duration   15–16
  management of heart attacks   12–16
hyperlipidaemia   35–6
  correction   65
  enhancing smoking effects   39
  in stable angina   94
  management   45
  see also cholesterol levels
hypertension
  control   30
    benefits   37, 104
    by drugs   37–8
    in secondary CHD prevention   51
    non-pharmacological   37
  reduced incidence   28
  reduction   21

risk factor in CHD   2, 36–8, 63
  self-management   49
hyperventilation   86

indomethacin   15
intermediate coronary syndrome   92
intraventricular septum rupture   15
isosorbide dinitrate   19, 108, 109
isosorbide mononitrate   19, 109

Judkins technique (angiography)   101
jugular venous pressure, during heart
    attack   6

left main stem stenosis   95–6, 97
left ventricular failure   52–3
life expectancy
  coronary artery disease   64
  factors influencing   63
lifestyle changes   29
  in secondary CHD prevention   50–1
lignocaine   10
lungs
  crepitations in bases   6
  pain, differential diagnosis   8

metoprolol   10, 111
mexiletine   21
mitral valve
  incompetence   61
  prolapse   86
  regurgitation   20
Moduretic   19
mortality rate, from heart attacks   2–3
  in early stages   3
mouth-to-mouth resuscitation   12
musculoskeletal pain   9, 86
myocardial infarction
  definition   1
  factors influencing recovery   62–3
  late complications   18–20
  life expectancy   63
  prognosis   63, 64–5
  rehabilitation   61–2
  ventricular extrasystoles   13
  see also heart attacks
myocardial rupture   15

nadolol   111
nifedipine   19, 113, 114
nitrates   108–10, 120–1
  combination therapy   114–15
nuclear imaging, for ischaemia   100–1
nurses, employed in general practice   43

obesity
  advice 106
  avoidance for well-being 105–6
  avoiding snacks 47
  control: in management of
      hypertension 37
    methods 40
  risk factor in CHD 2, 31, 39–40
  weight gain of ex-smokers 106
  weight reduction 21
occupational therapy 59
oesophageal pain 9, 86
oesophagitis 9
oxprenolol 111

pain
  angina differentiated from myocardial
      infarction 7–8
  functional 86
  in unstable angina 92
  musculoskeletal 9, 86
  oesophageal 9, 86
  of heart attack 5–6
  pericardial 8–9, 86
  pleuritic 8
  pulmonary 86
  see also chest pain
papillary muscle, rupture 15
percutaneous transluminal coronary
      angioplasty (PTCA) 23, 115–
      18
  compared with bypass surgery 116,
      118
  for unstable angina 121
pericarditis 86
  complication of heart attack 12
  differential diagnosis 8–9
  treatment 15
personality factors
  effect of beta-blockade 107
  in stress 40, 63
physical training see exercise training
physiotherapy 59
pindolol 110, 111
pleuritic pain 8
pneumothorax, chest pain 8
polyunsaturated fats 36
pre-infarction syndrome 92
preventive medicine 28
  GPs' role 32–4
  measures at population level 29–31
  patient compliance 47–9
  patient involvement 49

Prinzmetal's angina 92
propranolol 22, 111, 112
psychiatric treatment 66
psychological factors 60
  disabling effect 66
pulmonary embolism
  chest pain 8
  complication of heart attack 12
pulmonary oedema
  management 10
  treatment 14
pulse rate
  in cardiac arrest 11
  in heart attack 6

rehabilitation
  definition 59
  in cardiac disease 59–60
    methods 61–2
    objectives 60–1
    reducing risk of recurrence 61
  motivations 78
  Selly Oak hospital scheme 75–81
  see also exercise training
relaxation techniques, in control of
      hypertension 37
risk factors 2
  see also cholesterol levels;
      hypertension; obesity; smoking
Royal College of General Practitioners,
      initiatives in health care 27

salt
  in family diet 47
  intake reduction 29–30, 37
saturated fats in diet 35–6, 52
Scottish Health Education Group,
      address 57
screening
  benefits 104
  for angina 98–9
  for risk factors in CHD 44–5
Selly Oak rehabilitation scheme 75–81
sexual activity
  advice 107–8
  resumption 79
smoking
  as risk factor 2, 38–9, 63
  mechanisms stimulated 38–9, 105
  stopping: as preventive measure 21,
      50–1, 30
    effect on risk 105
    GPs' role 32–3
    to stop progress of CHD 65

social factors   67
sodium nitroprusside   14
Sones technique (angiography)   101
sotalol   111
streptokinase   23
stress
　advice   107
　avoidance, in hypertension
　　control   37
　in Type A personality   40, 63
　risk factor in CHD   40
stroke, reduced incidence   28
sulfinpyrazone   53
Swan Ganz technique   14
sweating, in heart attack   6
syncope, in heart attack   6

tachycardia
　in heart attack   6
　management   10
　treatment   20
technetium-99 imaging   101
thallium-201 imaging   101
thrombolysis   22–3
timolol   19, 22, 111
tissue plasminogen activators   23
treadmill testing   17, 68
　accuracy   100
　demonstrating patient's
　　capabilities   107
　for over-40-year-olds   98
　see also exercise testing

valve replacement, use of exercise
　　training   81
vasodilators, in heart failure
　　treatment   14
venous thrombosis
　complication of heart attack   12
　treatment   14–15
ventricular aneurysm   20, 61
ventricular extrasystoles   13
ventricular fibrillation   21
　from exercise testing   100
ventricular pressure, measurement   14
ventricular septal defect   20, 61
verapamil   20, 113, 121
visual aids   46
vomiting
　in heart attack   6
　in oesophagitis   9

Warfarin   21
weight checks   44
　see also obesity
weight training   80–1

xanthelasma   94
xanthomas, in hyperlipidaemia   94

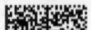